NEUROLOGY
FOR THE
PSYCHIATRY
SPECIALTY
BOARD
REVIEW,
Second Edition

BRUNNER/MAZEL CONTINUING EDUCATION IN PSYCHIATRY AND PSYCHOLOGY SERIES

Series Editor: Gene Usdin, M.D.

This series provides comprehensive, state-of-the-art study guides to help those who are preparing for advanced examinations in psychiatry and psychology. Written by experts representing various areas of specialization, the guides are designed to be accurate, current, and accessible.

*Software version also available. See the back of this book for a complete description and ordering information.

Brunner/Mazel Continuing Education in Psychiatry Series No. 7

NEUROLOGY FOR THE PSYCHIATRY SPECIALTY BOARD REVIEW, Second Edition

Leon A. Weisberg, M.D.

Professor of Neurology
Head of Neurology
Vice Chairman, Department of Psychiatry and Neurology
Tulane University School of Medicine
New Orleans, Louisiana

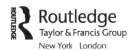

Routledge
Taylor & Francis Group
New York   London

First published 1998 by BRUNNER\MAZEL, INC.

This edition published 2013 by Routledge
711 Third Avenue, New York, NY 10017
27 Church Road, Hove East Sussex BN3 2FA

Routledge is an imprint of the Taylor & Francis Group, an informa business

NEUROLOGY FOR THE PSYCHIATRY SPECIALTY BOARD REVIEW, Second Edition

This book was set in Times Roman. The editors were Heather Worley and Lynne Lackenbach.

A CIP catalog record for this book is available from the British Library.

Library of Congress Cataloging-in-Publication Data

Weisberg, Leon A., 1941–
    Neurology for the psychiatry specialty board review/Leon A.
Weisberg. — 2nd ed.
        p.   cm. — (Brunner/Mazel continuing education in psychiatry
and psychology series no. 7)
    Includes bibliographical references.

    1. Neurology—Examinations, questions, etc.   I. Title.
II. Series.
    [DNLM: 1. Neurology—examination questions.   2. Psychiatry—
examination questions.   WL 18.2 W426n 1998]
RC343.5.W45   1998
616.8'0076—DC21
DNLM/DLC
for Library of Congress   97-36014
                                                                       CIP

ISBN 0-87630-868-X

CONTENTS

FOREWORD

Dr. Leon Weisberg is an outstanding educator, clinician and researcher in the field of neurology, especially as it pertains to psychiatry. As professor and head of neurology and vice-chair in the only joint department of psychiatry and neurology in the country, Tulane University School of Medicine, he is especially qualified to consider the necessary information about neurology that graduates of training programs should be familiar with as it relates to psychiatry.

The first edition of this book, published in 1992, was highly successful, serving as an important source for many candidates taking their boards in psychiatry and neurology as well as for those practitioners wanting a review of neurology as it pertains to psychiatry. To Weisberg's credit, he did not just add a few topics or concepts to the original edition, but has accomplished a major revision. He has included many new pertinent topics in his second edition by incorporating the latest material and knowledge. From a stylistic viewpoint, he has included a varied testing format, adding clinical vignettes and matching true-false questions to the multiple-choice format of the first edition. Weisberg has made it easier for readers by reducing the reference volumes from 17 to 6. He had many carefully chosen colleagues review the volume.

For me, one who stopped examining for the boards years ago, this volume is a helpful reminder of much of what current trainees are being taught and what clinicians and educators should know in their practice.

GENE USDIN, M.D.
Clinical Professor Emeritus of Psychiatry
Louisiana State University School of Medicine
New Orleans, Louisiana
Past President, American College of Psychiatrists

PREFACE

This book was prepared as a supplement and update to the first edition. The topics chosen are the most frequently encountered in clinical neurology and neurosciences. In the first edition, all questions were of multiple-choice format and based on factual knowledge and information. In this text, emphasis is on a varied testing format—including clinical vignettes, matching, true–false, and multiple-choice questions. All these types of questions are likely to be encountered on board certification and recertification examinations as well as on the in-service examination in both psychiatry and neurology.

The topics chosen for analysis complement those in the first edition. A certain amount of redundancy of material is to be expected; however, almost none of the questions in this edition are identical to those in the first edition. In addition, emphasis is placed on new material and knowledge not available at the time of writing of the first edition. For each question and answer, an explanation is referenced to standard textbooks which should be available in most medical libraries and bookstores. Maximal benefit for utilization of this book is obtained by initially reviewing the material in one or more of the standard textbooks and then attempting to answer questions on each topic. If areas of weakness are identified, the reader should refer back to the textbook to fill any gaps in knowledge identified by incorrect responses. In contrast to the first edition, which referenced 17 standard textbooks, this edition references six standard textbooks. The smaller number of reference books makes it easier for the reader to check sources. I utilized standard "encyclopedic" references as well as general neurology textbooks which can be reviewed quickly. For obvious reasons, *Essentials of Clinical Neurology,* written by this author, is my favorite, and I consider it the best general reference for clinical neurology.

After the questions and answers were prepared, they were reviewed by medical students, house officers (psychiatry, neurology), and faculty (psychiatry, neurology, neuroscience) in our combined Department of Psychiatry and Neurology at Tulane Medical School. This was done to identify voids in knowledge by this author as well as to clarify any vagueness in the questions and explanations.

Once again, in preparing this neurology review, I recognized certain embarrassing voids in my understanding of neurology and preparing this text has served as an excellent review and learning device for me. I wish you, the reader, the best in your examination preparation process, and I hope this book will be of assistance in passing your examination.

LEON A. WEISBERG

REFERENCES

> **Note:** With dramatic advances continually being made in the clinical sciences, it is a challenge for physicians to keep abreast of both modifications in treatment that such advances require and of new drugs being introduced each year. The author and publisher of this volume have taken care to make certain that the doses of drugs and schedules of treatment are correct and compatible with the standards generally accepted at the time of publication. However, it is essential for the reader to become fully cognizant of the information in the instruction inserts provided with each drug or therapeutic agent prior to administration or prescription.
>
> Further, as some of the topics are by nature ambiguous, it is suggested that the reader consult the indicated reference sources for clarification should there be a discrepancy between the answer selected and that which appears in the book.

Each question, answer, and explanation is referenced to a current, standard neurology textbook, and/or journal article. The textbooks are assigned numbers here, and these numbers are utilized throughout the text. When journal publications are used, the journal title is given, together with the volume and page numbers and year, so that the article can be found in the library. The reader is introduced to several types of standard neurology textbooks, including the encyclopedic type of reference, as well as the briefer review. The former is more appropriate in reviewing a specific topic and the latter as a review for a Board or in-service examination.

1. L. P. Rowland (Ed.), *Merritt's Textbook of Neurology* (9th ed.). Williams & Wilkins, Baltimore, 1995.
2. L. A. Weisberg, R. L. Strub, and C. A. Garcia, *Essentials of Clinical Neurology* (3rd ed.). Mosby, Philadelphia, 1996.
3. W. Demyer, *Technique of the Neurological Examination* (4th ed.). McGraw-Hill, New York, 1994.
4. L. A. Weisberg, R. L. Strub, and C. A. Garcia, *Decision Making in Adult Neurology* (2nd ed.). D. C. Decker, Toronto, 1993.
5. J. O. Greenberg. Neuroimaging—*Principles of Neurology*. McGraw-Hill, New York, 1995.
6. B. F. Westmoreland, E. E. Benarroch, and J. R. Daube. *Medical Neurosciences.* Little, Brown, Boston, 1994.

1

NEUROANATOMY

Match the area of the nervous system involved with the clinical findings given, using answers A–Z. Each item may be used once, more than once, or not at all.

Matching Localization

A.	Left occipital lobe	N.	Neuromuscular junction
B.	Right parietal lobe	O.	Anterior horn cell
C.	Right temporal lobe	P.	Dorsal midbrain
D.	Left temporal lobe	Q.	Dorsal column
E.	Frontal lobe	R.	Lateral medulla
F.	Left internal capsule	S.	Left pons
G.	Left thalamus	T.	Left facial nerve
H.	Oculomotor nerve	U.	T9-10 disk
I.	Peroneal nerve	V.	L3-L4 disk
J.	Median nerve	W.	Cauda equina
K.	Ulnar nerve	X.	Vagus nerve
L.	L5 root	Y.	Spinal accessory nerve
M.	C5 root	Z.	Cavernous sinus

1. _____ Apathy, abulia, gait apraxia, incontinence.

2. _____ Inability to dress self, neglect of contralateral half of body.

3. _____ Intermittent extremity weakness and double vision.

4. _____ Weakness of dorsiflexion and eversion of foot.

5. _____ Inability to close left eye, smile pulled to right, difficulty looking to left, and hemiparesis.

6. _____ Loss of sensation of right face, arm, and leg.

7. _____ Bilateral leg weakness, incontinence, spasticity, numbness from lower trunk downward, and positive Babinski signs.

8. _____ Vertigo, ataxia of right side, loss of pain sensation on left side, and difficulty swallowing.

9. _____ Loss of sensation of right upper face, diplopia.

10. _____ Inability to adduct fingers, with a "claw-hand" deformity and sensory loss involving fourth and fifth digits.

11. _____ Right homonymous hemianopsia.

12. _____ Weakness and fasciculations.

13. _____ Confusion and left superior homonymous quadrantanopia.

14. _____ Wernicke aphasia and right homonymous hemianopsia.

15. _____ Right-sided weakness involving face, arm, and leg.

16. _____ Bilateral leg weakness which is more severe on left side, urinary incontinence, diminished ankle and knee reflexes, plantar flexor responses.

17. _____ Dysphonia and dysphagia.

18. _____ Weakness of orbicularis oculi, buccinators, and platysma muscles.

19. _____ Numbness of thumb and weakness in thumb flexion with normal upper extremity reflexes.

20. _____ Weakness of dorsiflexion of big toe with normal strength of foot.

Match major neurotransmitters with the region of the brain which is the source of these chemical substances.

A. Norepinephrine
B. Dopamine
C. Serotonin
D. Acetylcholine

21. _____ Locus ceruleus of upper pons.

22. _____ Substantia nigra and ventral tegmentum of midbrain.

23. _____ Dorsal raphe of posterior midbrain.

24. _____ Nucleus basalis of Meynert in frontal lobes.

Match the neuropsychological dysfunction with the lobe of the brain.

A. Receptive aphasia
B. Amnesia
C. Gerstmann syndrome

    D.   Anosognosia of Babinski
    E.   Akinetic mutism

25. _____ Left superior-posterior temporal lobe.

26. _____ Temporal lobes.

27. _____ Supramarginal and angular gyrus.

28. _____ Frontal lobes.

29. _____ Right parietal lobe.

Match the neurological feature with the brain location.

    A.   Involved in negative symptoms of schizophrenia; prominent dopaminergic pathway; lesions of this region may cause depression.
    B.   Sylvian fissure separates from frontal and parietal lobe; common site of origin of partial complex seizures.
    C.   Involves Papez system; part of olfactory system; injury may cause Kluver-Bucy syndrome.
    D.   Lesions may cause astereognosia, graphesthesia, agraphia, acalculia.
    E.   Visual, auditory, sensory relay nuclei.

30. _____ Thalamus.

31. _____ Parietal lobe.

32. _____ Temporal lobe.

33. _____ Dorsolateral prefrontal cortex.

34. _____ Limbic lobe.

Match the visual loss pattern with the site in the visual pathway.

    A.   Monocular centrocecal scotoma.
    B.   Bitemporal hemianopsia.
    C.   Superior homonymous quadrantanopia.
    D.   Inferior homonymous quadrantanopia.
    E.   Homonymous hemianopsia with macular sparing.

35. _____ Optic nerve.

36. _____ Occipital lobe.

37. _____ Parietal lobe.

38. _____ Temporal lobe.

39. _____ Optic chiasm.

Match the clinical findings with the brainstem localization.

    A.   Ipsilateral facial and abducens paresis and contralateral hemiparesis.
    B.   Ipsilateral gaze and abducens paresis; contralateral hemiparesis.
    C.   Ipsilateral oculomotor paresis and contralateral hemiparesis.
    D.   Drop attacks and quadriplegia with intact consciousness and normal eye movements.
    E.   Ipsilateral oculomotor paresis; contralateral intention tremor and hemiataxia.

40. _____ Caudal ventral paramedian pontine (Millard-Gubler syndrome).

41. _____ Paramedian pontine (Foville syndrome).

42. _____ Middle medial midbrain (Weber syndrome).

43. _____ Bilateral ventral pontine (locked-in syndrome).

44. _____ Ventral rostral midbrain (Claude syndrome).

Match the clinical finding with the vascular occlusive ischemic syndrome.

    A.   Nonfluent aphasia; right hemiparesis involving face and arm.
    B.   Right leg weakness and anesthesia.
    C.   Right homonymous hemianopsia.
    D.   Right pure motor hemiparesis.
    E.   Dysarthria—clumsy hand syndrome.

45. _____ Left middle cerebral artery (MCA) syndrome.

46. _____ Left lenticulostriate artery syndrome.

47. _____ Left anterior cerebral artery (ACA) syndrome.

48. _____ Right posterior cerebral artery (PCA) syndrome.

49. _____ Pontine lacunar syndrome.

RESPONSES AND EXPLANATIONS

1. **E.** The frontal lobe includes primary motor cortex, frontal eye fields, motor speech (Broca) area, dorsolateral prefrontal cortex (involved in attention, memory, motor planning), orbitofrontal, and medial prefrontal regions (involved in emotional behavior). Gait apraxia and incontinence are due to medial frontal motor involvement; apathy and abulia are due to dorsolateral prefrontal involvement. *(Ref. 6, pp. 496–498)*

2. **B.** The parietal lobe is involved in somatosensory and visual-spatial information processing. It includes somatosensory cortex in the postcentral gyrus. Lesions in this location may cause impairment of two-point discrimination, joint position sensibility, and touch localization. Lesions on the right parietal cortex may cause sensory neglect of the left side of the body and dressing apraxia. *(Ref. 6, p. 497)*

3. **N.** Disorders of the neuromuscular junction cause fluctuating levels of weakness with fatigue on sustained exertion. Myasthenia gravis is the characteristic disorder and may initially involve extraocular muscles (resulting in diplopia) and levator palpebral muscles (resulting in ptosis). It is the *fluctuating* weakness which differentiates myasthenia gravis from other muscle or nerve diseases. *(Ref. 2, pp. 526–532; Ref. 6, pp. 357–358)*

4. **I.** The peroneal nerve supplies the anterior tibialis and evertors of the foot. Injury to this nerve should be differentiated from L-4 (quadriceps weakness) and L-5 (extensor hallucis longus weakness plus some foot extension weakness) radiculopathy. In lumbar radiculopathy, patients report back pain, and this is not present in peroneal neuropathy. The common peroneal nerve is frequently subject to injury secondary to leg trauma, as it is superficial and in close relationship to the head and neck of the fibula. The peroneal nerve may also be injured by compression behind the knee, as occurs with prolonged kneel-cross position. *(Ref. 6, pp. 343, 346)*

5. **S.** A paramedian pontine lesion including facial nerve nucleus and medial longitudinal fasciculus would explain these findings. If the ventral pons is involved, hemiparesis occurs due to involvement of the corticospinal tract. *(Ref. 1, p. 249; Ref. 6, p. 451)*

6. **G.** The thalamus relays information for the sensory, motor, consciousness (ascending reticular activating system), and limbic systems. The ventral posterior nuclei relay information to the somatosensory cortex of the parietal lobe. The ventral posterior thalamic nuclei are the termination of the spinothalamic and medial lemniscal pathways. *(Ref. 6, pp. 464–466)*

7. **U.** Paraparesis with midthoracic sensory disturbance and incontinence indicates spinal cord compression in the thoracic region. *(Ref. 6, pp. 370, 396)*

8. **R.** The lateral medulla and cerebellum are supplied by the posterior inferior cerebellar artery. Infarction in this territory causes Wallenberg syndrome with dysarthria and dysphagia due to nucleus ambiguous involvement, ipsilateral facial loss of pain and temperature due to involvement of the descending trigeminal tract, contralateral pain and temperature impairment due to spinothalamic tract involvement, Horner's syndrome due to descending sympathetic involvement, ataxia due to involvement of the inferior cerebellar peduncle, vertigo due to vestibular system involvement. *(Ref. 1, p. 249; Ref. 6, p. 453)*

9. **Z.** The cavernous sinus is situated on either side of the pituitary fossa. It contains the internal carotid artery, cranial nerves III, IV, and VI (extraocular nerves which may cause diplopia), and the ophthalmic sensory branch of the trigeminal nerve (causes facial numbness). *(Ref. 6, p. 282)*

10. **K.** The ulnar nerve supplies the intrinsic hand muscles and sensation to the fourth and fifth fingers. Weakness of the intrinsic hand muscles leads to claw hand deformity and guttering appearance due to adductor muscles which are weak and wasted. *(Ref. 6, pp. 342, 344, 346)*

11. **A.** The occipital cortex includes the primary visual region located along the calcarine fissure on the medial occipital lobe (area 17). This causes homonymous hemianopsia with macular region sparing. Lesions may also cause scintillating scotomas, visual hallucinations, and illusions (macropsia, micropsia, achromatopsia in which objects lack color). *(Ref. 6, pp. 497, 508)*

12. **O.** Anterior horn cells represent lower motor neurons. When affected, weakness with atrophy and wasting occur initially in distal distribution. Weakness may then proceed to proximal distribution. The presence of fasciculations indicates denervation. *(Ref. 6, pp. 201, 240, 340, 355)*

13. **C.** The temporal lobe includes the primary auditory cortex, the auditory and visual association cortex, and part of the limbic lobe. Receptive aphasia occurs with dominant temporal lesions, and confusion occurs with nondominant lesions. Optic radiations pass through the temporal lobe to cause superior quadrant visual field defect. *(Ref. 6, pp. 485, 498)*

14. **D.** With dominant temporal lesion, receptive comprehensive (Wernicke) aphasia and right-sided visual field defect occur. There is *no* associated hemiparesis. *(Ref. 6, pp. 490–491)*

15. **F.** Pure motor hemiparesis is due to either internal capsule or ventral pontine lesion. Capsular lesions are usually due to lenticulostriate arteriolar infarction which results from chronic hypertensive disease. Motor fibers are localized within the *genu* of the internal capsule. *(Ref. 2, pp. 282–283)*

16. **W.** The cauda equina comprises multiple nerve roots derived from the lower portion of the spinal cord. These represent the lumbar and sacral regions. Motor and sensory involvement are frequently *asymmetric*. There is usually bladder disturbance. *(Ref. 6, p. 396)*

17. **X.** The vagus is a mixed nerve which innervates the striated muscle of the soft palate, pharynx, and larynx to cause difficulty swallowing and speaking. *(Ref. 6, p. 415)*

18. **T.** With facial nerve involvement, there is weakness of the muscles of facial expression in both the upper and lower face. There may be loss of taste on the anterior two-thirds of the tongue. With cortical lesions, the upper face is spared. *(Ref. 6, p. 422)*

19. **J.** With median nerve lesion, there is weakness of thumb flexion and thumb region numbness. The median nerve is compressed at the wrist in carpal tunnel syndrome, and there is positive Tinel and Phalen signs. With C-7 radiculopathy, the triceps muscle is weak and the triceps reflex is diminished. *(Ref. 2, pp. 163, 467)*

20. **L.** With L-5 radiculopathy, there is weakness of the extensor hallucis longus (the big toe dorsiflexor), with normal strength for plantar flexion (gastrocnemius, which is S-1 innervated). The anterior tibialis is innervated by both L-4 and L-5 equally and is not weak with *only* L-5 radiculopathy even though there may be *electrical* evidence (EMG) of L-5 involvement. With peroneal nerve palsy, dorsiflexion of the foot (foot drop) is most prominent. *(Ref. 2, pp. 596–597)*

21. **A**
22. **B**
23. **C**
24. **D**

21–24. Norepinephrine cells are located in the locus ceruleus of the upper pons and the lower midbrain and send projections to areas that mediate sensory stimulation responses (thalamus, basal forebrain, cerebral cortex). They are important in maintaining attention and wakefulness. Dopaminergic neurons are located in the substantia nigra, and dopamine is deficient in Parkinson's disease. Serotonergic neurons from the raphe nucleus modulate non-REM sleep. Cholinergic neurons of the basal forebrain modulate arousal, wakefulness, learning, and memory. Their deficiency may explain certain of the cognitive-behavioral disturbances of Alzheimer's disease. *(Ref. 6, pp. 311–320)*

25. **A**
26. **B**
27. **C**
28. **E**
29. **D**

25–29. The primary auditory cortex (areas 41 and 42) in the superior temporal gyrus (Heschl gyrus) receives auditory input from the medial geniculate body (the auditory portion of the thalamus). Lesions cause Wernicke aphasia. Bilateral damage to the hippocampus, entorhinal cortex, mammillary bodies, and dorsomedial thalamus are involved in memory; lesions involving these structures cause amnesia. *Bilateral* medial temporal lobe lesions cause amnesia. Gerstmann syndrome includes right–left confusion, finger agnosia, agraphia, and acalculia. This is due to dominant inferior parietal (supramarginal and angular gyrus) lesions. Patients with right parietal lesions may show sensory neglect of the left hemibody and may show denial and inattention to motor deficit (anosognosia of Babinski). Patients with dorsolateral prefrontal lesions lack spontancity and show psychomotor slowing and may appear akinetic with lack of spontaneous speech. *(Ref. 6, pp. 496–499)*

30. **E**
31. **D**
32. **B**
33. **A**
34. **C**

30–34. The thalamus is part of the diencephalon. It contains nuclei within the third ventricular wall which relay information involving the sensory, motor, consciousness, and limbic systems. The parietal lobe processes somatosensory and visual information. The temporal lobe is usually the site of psychomotor (partial complex) seizures. The dorsolateral prefrontal cortex is involved in attention, memory, and motor planning, and patients with lesions in this region show lack of spontaneity and psychomotor retardation. *(Ref. 6, pp. 466–467, 496–499)*

35. **A**
36. **E**
37. **D**
38. **C**
39. **B**

35–39. Lesions of the optic nerve cause unilateral visual disturbances with reduced visual acuity and impaired color vision and scotoma (an island of blindness surrounding a sea of vision). Pupils are equal in size but the involved pupil does not respond well to direct light stimulation. Funduscopy shows disk margin blurring and later, optic atrophy. With occipital lobe lesions, there is homonymous hemianopsia with or without macular sparing. Pupillary response and funduscopic exam are normal. With parietal lesions, upper visual field fibers which represent the lower visual field are affected, causing inferior homonymous quadrantanopia; whereas with temporal lesions, lower fibers are affected, causing superior homonymous quadrantanopia. Remember that everything is *reversed* in the visual system such that *upper* visual fibers represent *lower* visual fields. With optic chiasmal lesions, crossing visual fibers which represent temporal visual fields are affected, causing bitemporal hemianopsia. *(Ref. 2, pp. 199–204)*

40. A
41. B
42. C
43. D
44. E

40–44. With caudal ventral paramedian pontine ischemic brain stem lesions, there is ipsilateral facial and abducens paresis with contralateral hemiparesis. With paramedian pontine lesions, there is ipsilateral gaze and abducens paresis and contralateral hemiparesis but no facial weakness. With ventral midbrain lesions, there is ipsilateral oculomotor paresis and contralateral hemiparesis. With midbrain lesions involving the tegmentum, red nucleus, cerebellar peduncle, and oculomotor nerve nucleus, there is ipsilateral oculomotor paresis and contralateral hemiataxia and intention tremor. If there is bilateral ventral pontine involvement, sudden episodes of falling, referred to as "drop attacks," may occur. There may be gradriplegia with normal consciousness and eye movements (locked-in syndrome) due to sparing of dorsal pons. It is important to know brainstem anatomy involving the midbrain, pons, and medulla, and to know whether neural structures are located medially or laterally, ventral or dorsal. *(Ref. 1, p. 249; Ref. 2, pp. 276–277; Ref. 6, p. 451)*

45. A
46. D
47. B
48. C
49. E

45–49. With left MCA ischemic syndrome, the dominant hemisphere is involved, causing aphasia. When there is expressive aphasia, there is usually accompanying hemiparesis, whereas if aphasia is receptive type, there is no hemiparesis. With MCA ischemia, the motor cortex supplying the face and arm are involved, whereas leg fibers which are located on the medial surface of the hemisphere supplied by ACA are spared. With ACA ischemia, the leg is weak and numb but the face and arm are not involved. With lenticulostriate artery occlusion, there is ischemia of the internal capsule, causing pure motor hemiparesis. With small vessel disease involving brainstem and specifically causing ischemia in the ventral pons, dysarthria and clumsiness in one hand may develop. With PCA ischemia, contralateral visual disturbance consisting of homonymous hemianopsia may be the only neurological disturbance. *(Ref. 2, pp. 270–276)*

2

NEUROLOGICAL LOCALIZATION AND EXAMINATION

True or False

1. _____ Polyneuropathy usually causes acral weakness and paresthesias, and initial symptoms occur in hands.

2. _____ Myopathy initially causes difficulty climbing stairs and arising from a chair; swallowing and speech disturbances and problems supporting the head may occur.

3. _____ Fasciculations are seen in patients with motor neuron disease but may also be seen in normal subjects.

4. _____ Alzheimer's disease patients have prominent memory and cognitive impairment, and rarely show motor or gait impairment.

5. _____ Aphasia and chorea are seen in patients with right hemispheric dysfunction.

6. _____ When papilledema develops, blind spots increase in size.

7. _____ Positive Babinski sign indicates upper motor neuron lesion in both children and adults.

8. _____ Spasticity, rigidity, and contractures are all manifestations of parkinsonism.

9. _____ Ataxia and dysmetria are signs of cerebellar dysfunction.

10. _____ In amyotrophic lateral sclerosis (ALS), there are both upper and lower motor neuron abnormalities affecting arms and legs, as well as swallowing difficulties and diplopia.

11. _____ Dysarthria and aphasia are synonymous terms indicating abnormal language communication.

12. _____ Ptosis is due to weakness of the levator palpebral muscle.

13. _____ C-5 sensory dermatome includes the lateral aspect of the upper arm.

14. _____ Sensory distribution of the lateral femoral cutaneous nerve includes the upper thigh and the perineal (saddle) region.

15. _____ When focusing on a near object, major motor activities occur in both medial recti; whereas when focusing on a far object, major motor activities occur in lateral recti.

16. _____ In patients with Adie's (myotonic) pupil response, pupils are dilated and have slow response to light and accommodation.

17. _____ In patients with Argyll-Robertson syndrome, pupils are miotic, irregular in size, accommodate normally, but react poorly to light.

18. _____ In diabetic patients who develop ischemic oculomotor paresis, the involved pupil does not respond to light and is maximally dilated.

19. _____ In patients with left-sided medial longitudinal fasciculus (MLF) lesion, diplopia would occur upon gazing to the left only.

20. _____ In patients with Bell's palsy, the frontalis, orbicularis oculi, buccinator, and platysma muscles are weak.

Multiple Choice

Choose the appropriate response.

21. _____ Clinical features of pseudobulbar palsy:

   A. Dysarthria
   B. Dysphagia
   C. Emotional lability
   D. Hyperactive jaw reflex
   E. All of the above

22. _____ The major abnormality(ies) of reflexes:

   A. Asymmetry
   B. Unsustained clonus

C. Positive Hoffman sign
D. Pendularity
E. All of the above

23. _____ In a patient with mild myopathy, reflexes would be:

A. Increased
B. Decreased
C. Normal
D. Show Babinski sign
E. Show clonus

24. _____ Clinical features of upper motor neuron lesion:

A. Extensor plantar response
B. Absent abdominal-cremasteric reflexes
C. Clasp-knife spasticity
D. Clonus
E. All of the above

A 49-year-old alcoholic man who smokes heavily develops difficulty walking. Examination shows ataxic gait with impaired tandem walking and negative Romberg sign. He has normal finger-to-nose movement but impaired heel-to-shin maneuver, absent ankle jerks, impaired vibration sensation at the toes but normal proprioception.

25. _____ What is the most likely neurological mechanism for difficulty walking?

A. Peripheral neuropathy
B. Carcinomatous cerebellar degeneration
C. Alcoholic vermis cerebellar atrophy
D. Guillain-Barré syndrome
E. Myasthenic syndrome

26. _____ Which diagnostic test is most likely to help establish the diagnosis in this case?

A. EMG/NCV
B. LP
C. Tensilon test
D. CT with contrast
E. Noncontrast MRI

27. _____ Anisocoria may be due to:

A. Horner syndrome
B. Metabolic encephalopathy
C. 1% pilocarpine eye drops instilled in both eyes
D. Diabetic mononeuropathy
E. All of the above

28. _____ The following is manifestation of corticospinal tract (CST) lesion:

A. Weakness, hypotonia, Babinski sign
B. Weakness and rigidity
C. Weakness and apraxia
D. Spasticity
E. Parkinsonism

29. _____ To classify aphasia, test the following function(s):

A. Reading
B. Writing
C. Memory
D. Spontaneous speech
E. All of the above

30. _____ The earliest visualized funduscopic finding of papilledema:

A. Blurred disk margins
B. Retinal hemorrhages
C. Exudates
D. Pericapillary sheathing
E. Loss of spontaneous venous pulsations

31. _____ A 60-year-old hypertensive diabetic develops horizontal (far gaze) diplopia, right facial weakness, and left hemiplegia. A neurological lesion would be most likely located in this region:

A. Pons
B. Medulla
C. Midbrain
D. Right internal capsule
E. Right thalamus

32. _____ Gerstmann syndrome includes:

A. Right–left confusion
B. Finger agnosia
C. Agraphia
D. Acalculia
E. All of the above

33. _____ Anton syndrome involves:

A. Anomia
B. Amnesia
C. Denial of blindness
D. Gait apraxia
E. Anosognosia

34. _____ Palatal myoclonus is associated with lesion in this region:

A. Subthalamus
B. Thalamus
C. Inferior olivary nucleus
D. Parietal lobe
E. Broca region

35. _____ If a patient has been diagnosed as "locked in," the following structures are likely affected:

   A. Optic radiation
   B. Ascending reticular activating formation
   C. Corticospinal and corticobulbar tracts
   D. Medial longitudinal fasciculus
   E. None of the above

36. _____ A 68-year-old hypertensive man awakens with uncontrolled flailing movements of the left arm and leg. CT/MRI will most likely show lesion in this location:

   A. Right subthalamus
   B. Right thalamus
   C. Left putamen
   D. Right internal capsule
   E. Left cerebellar hemisphere

37. _____ A finding of wide-based slapping gait suggests this diagnosis:

   A. Tabes dorsalis
   B. Bilateral peroneal nerve palsies
   C. Cerebral palsy
   D. Cerebellar ataxia
   E. Wernicke encephalopathy

38. _____ Clinical features of cerebellar lesion:

   A. Overshooting of target on motor movement
   B. Impaired rapid alternating movements
   C. Hypotonia
   D. Nystagmus
   E. All of the above

39. _____ A flail-foot is characteristic of this condition:

   A. Diabetic neuropathy
   B. Sciatic nerve injury
   C. Spinal cord lesion
   D. Peroneal nerve injury
   E. Normal-pressure hydrocephalus

40. _____ Components of the Glasgow coma scale:

   A. Eye opening, verbal response, motor response
   B. Level of consciousness, pupillary response, motor response
   C. Memory, level of consciousness
   D. Language, speech, memory
   E. None of the above

41. _____ An intramuscular injection in the lower medial quadrant of the buttock might cause weakness of this muscle:

   A. Anterior tibialis
   B. Gastrocnemius
   C. Posterior tibialis
   D. Peroneus longus
   E. All of the above

42. _____ Finding of left oculomotor dysfunction and right hemiparesis is caused by lesion in this region:

   A. Left midbrain
   B. Right pontine
   C. Left thalamic
   D. Right midbrain
   E. Right internal capsule

43. _____ Corticospinal fibers are located in this portion of the internal capsule.

   A. Anterior
   B. Genu
   C. Posterior
   D. Retrolenticular
   E. None of the above

44. _____ Alexia without agraphia may be associated with:

   A. Right homonymous hemianopsia
   B. Finger agnosia
   C. Right–left confusion
   D. Acalculia
   E. Gait apraxia

Matching

Match the examination finding with the clinical neurological disorder.

   A. Shawl-like sensory impairment; wasted, weak, fasciculating hand muscles
   B. Wasting, fasciculation, weakness, bilateral Babinski signs, hyperreflexia
   C. Gait apraxia
   D. Crossed analgesia involving ipsilateral face and contralateral arm, trunk, and leg
   E. Saddle sparing sensory impairment in patient with mid-thoracic sensory anesthesia and spastic paraparesis

45. _____ Normal-pressure hydrocephalus (NPH)

46. _____ Amyotrophic lateral sclerosis (ALS)

47. _____ Syringomyelia

48. _____ Intradural intramedullary thoracic spinal cord neoplasm

49. _____ Pontine glioma

Match the motor activity with the appropriate innervation.

    A.   Flexion of forearm
    B.   Extension of forearm; wrist extension
    C.   Flexion of thumb; pronation of forearm
    D.   Adduction of fingers
    E.   Hip flexion; knee extension
    F.   Dorsiflexion and eversion of foot

50. _____ Peroneal nerve

51. _____ Medial nerve

52. _____ Radial nerve

53. _____ Femoral nerve

54. _____ Musculocutaneous nerve

55. _____ Ulnar nerve

Match the muscle stretch (deep) reflex with the appropriate nerve roots.

    A.   Jaw jerk
    B.   Biceps reflex
    C.   Triceps reflex
    D.   Knee reflex
    E.   Ankle reflex
    F.   Abdominal reflex
    G.   Cremasteric reflex

56. _____ C-5 and C-6

57. _____ Trigeminal nerve

58. _____ C-7 and C-8

59. _____ S-1 and S-2

60. _____ L-3 and L-4

61. _____ L-1 and L-2

62. _____ T-8 and T-12

RESPONSES AND EXPLANATIONS

1. **F.** Peripheral polyneuropathy causes extremity (acral) motor (weakness) and sensory (paresthesias, numbness) symptoms and signs; however, the *longest* nerves are initially affected. This means that initial clinical manifestations will be in the *feet and legs,* before the fingers and hands are involved. If initial clinical manifestations occur in the hands without lower extremity involvement, consider focal compressive neuropathy, e.g., carpal tunnel syndrome. *(Ref. 3, pp. 230–235)*

2. **T.** Polymyopathy initially causes proximal distribution weakness. Pelvic-girdle hip weakness is the initial disturbance, and then shoulder–upper arm weakness develops. Bulbar muscle involvement may cause dysphagia and dysarthria. Neck muscle weakness is seen in myopathies. Early-onset ptosis and diplopia are highly suggestive of myasthenia gravis. *(Ref. 2, pp. 143, 147; Ref. 3, p. 230)*

3. **T.** Fasciculations are spontaneous discharges of the motor units of all muscle fibers innervated by a single axon. They are of neuropathic origin and are due to anterior horn cell disease or spinal root involvement (radiculopathy). They may occur in normal subjects without accompanying wasting or weakness. *(Ref. 2, pp. 620–621; Ref. 3, pp. 233–235)*

4. **T.** Alzheimer's disease causes cognitive and behavioral disorders but does not usually affect motor function, gait, or balance. If the patient becomes demented and shows other neurological disturbances, consider an alternative cause for dementia: e.g., chorea—consider Huntington's disease; myoclonus—consider Creutzfeldt-Jakob disease. *(Ref. 2, pp. 413–417)*

5. **F.** Aphasia indicates dominant (left) hemispheric dysfunction. Chorea indicates subcortical basal ganglia (caudate) dysfunction. Right-hemispheric (nondominant) signs include inattention or neglect of left side of space. *(Ref. 2, pp. 421–424, 622–623; Ref. 3, pp. 80, 270)*

6. **T.** Papilledema is usually associated with no change in visual acuity or visual fields *except* for enlargement of blind spots. This can be detected by carefully performed visual field examination. Symptoms caused by papilledema due to increased intracranial pressure include transient visual obscurations and diplopia (due to lateral rectus dysfunction). *(Ref. 2, pp. 184–187)*

7. **F.** Positive Babinski sign may indicate incomplete corticospinal tract myelination in children less than 2 years of age and is a *normal* expected finding. In older children and adults, positive Babinski sign is *always* an abnormal neurological finding which demands explanation by neurodiagnostic studies. *(Ref. 2, pp. 34–35; Ref. 6, pp. 246–254)*

8. **F.** Rigidity is an increased resistance to passive movement (involving both agonists and antagonists). This is frequently associated with cogwheeling or ratcheting due to resting tremor superimposed on the rigidity. This is characteristic of parkinsonism. If the weak or paralyzed limb is not utilized, contractures or fixed joint deformities may develop. Spasticity is increased tone in antigravity muscles which occurs following corticospinal tract involvement, e.g., hemiplegia due to stroke. *(Ref. 2, pp. 626–627; Ref. 3, pp. 241–243)*

9. **T.** Ataxia (loss of coordination) and dysmetria (being off the mark or target) are both signs of cerebellar dysfunction. *(Ref. 6, pp. 298–290)*

10. **F.** In amyotrophic lateral sclerosis (ALS), there are extremity and bulbar signs of upper and lower motor neuron dysfunction. It is the dysphagia and respiratory disturbances which cause mortality in this disease. Abnormalities of eye movements leading to double vision do *not* occur in ALS. *(Ref. 2, pp. 488–492)*

11. **F.** Dysarthria is motor disorder of articulation. This may be due to dysfunction of cortical, subcortical, brainstem, or cerebellum structures. Aphasia represents language communication disorder such that abnormalities of spoken and written speech are equally impaired. With dysarthria, written speech will be entirely normal. *(Ref. 3, pp. 188–190)*

12. **T.** Ptosis or droopiness of eyelid is due to levator palpebral muscle weakness or to oculosympathetic paresis in Horner's syndrome. *(Ref. 3, pp. 150–152)*

13. **T.** C-5 sensory dermatome includes upper lateral arm and motor components including the biceps muscle and biceps reflex. It is important to understand the C-5, C-6, and C-7 radiculopathies in terms of sensory, motor, and reflex abnormalities caused by each root dysfunction. *(Ref. 3, pp. 223–226)*

14. **F.** Sensory distribution of the lateral femoral cutaneous nerve (derived from the upper lumbar roots) is the lateral upper thigh. The perianal or "saddle region" is supplied by sacral roots. This area is affected most commonly by spinal root or spinal cord lesions. Uncomfortable paresthesias involving the lateral thigh are called "meralgia paresthetica," and this disorder is commonly seen in diabetic neuropathy. *(Ref. 3, p. 373)*

15. **T.** With lateral rectus dysfunction, diplopia is maximal in far gaze, in which *divergence* occurs; whereas with medial rectus dysfunction, diplopia is maximal in near gaze, in which convergence occurs. With these extraocular disturbances, diplopia is horizontal. *(Ref. 3, pp. 114–117)*

16. **F.** Tonic (Adie pupil) shows absent constriction to light with slowed and tonic constriction to near target (accommodation). The pupil shows slow writhing movements when looked at with a slit lamp. Some patients report visual blurring due to pupillary light response abnormality. Adie syndrome occurs most commonly in young women and may be associated with absent deep tendon reflexes. There is rapid pupillary constriction following 0.125% pilocarpine, indicating denervation cholinergic sensitivity. *(Ref. 2, pp. 191–192; Ref. 3, pp. 149–150)*

17. **T.** In Argyll-Robertson pupillary syndrome, all these features are true; and this is *usually* but not always caused by neurosyphilis. *(Ref. 2, pp. 191–192; Ref. 3, pp. 149–150)*

18. **F.** In ischemic oculomotor paresis, the pupil is *usually* spared so that it is normal in size and reactivity. Pupillary fibers are located on the outside of nerves and are most sensitive to external compression (neoplasm, aneurysm, herniation syndrome), whereas extraocular and levator palpebrae fibers are internal and most sensitive to ischemia. *(Ref. 3, pp. 144–147, 430–431)*

19. **F.** In MLF lesions, there is internuclear ophthalmoplegia with medial rectus limitation ipsilateral to the side of the lesion, and there is horizontal nystagmus in the contralateral abducting eye. There is usually no diplopia, but if it occurs, it will usually occur upon looking to the right. Bilateral INO are most characteristic of brainstem lesions, especially *multiple sclerosis.* *(Ref. 2, pp. 195–196)*

20. **T.** In patients with Bell's palsy, muscles supplying both the upper and lower face are involved. Taste sensation on the anterior two-thirds of the tongue is impaired. Remember, platysma (shaving muscle) in the *neck* is innervated by facial nerves. *(Ref. 2, pp. 482–483; Ref. 3, pp. 318–321)*

21. **E.** There are reduced voluntary movements and spastic hyper-reflexia of the bulbar muscles, and the patient is unable to swallow normally. Speech is dysarthric due to bilateral corticobulbar involvement. There may be emotional lability (crying, laughing) with minimal or no provocation. Pseudobulbar palsy is caused by bilateral corticobulbar lesions (stroke, multiple sclerosis, ALS). Frontal release signs (snout, glabella) may be prominent. *(Ref. 2, p. 283; Ref. 3, pp. 185–186)*

22. **A.** The major reflex abnormalities are *asymmetry,* sustained *clonus,* and *Babinski sign.* All other findings may be seen in normal patients, *including* unsustained clonus or absent reflexes. *(Ref. 2, pp. 29–34; Ref. 3, pp. 245–246)*

23. **C.** In early or mild myopathy, reflexes may be normal. Reflexes are characteristically diminished in neuropathy and increased with upper motor neuron involvement. *(Ref. 2, pp. 41, 143, 147; Ref. 3, p. 232)*

24. **E.** All are features of upper motor neuron involvement. Extensor plantar response is Babinski sign. Remember, Hoffman reflex (finger and thumb flexion elicited by flicking the distal phalanx) is *not* the upper-extremity equivalent of Babinski sign. *(Ref. 2, pp. 488–492; Ref. 6, pp. 201–203)*

25. **C.** Alcoholic patients may develop cerebellar degeneration and nutritional deficiency polyneuropathy. With neuropathy, gait is impaired due to proprioception dysfunction, which is not present in this case because Romberg sign is negative. Gait disorder in this case is due to alcohol-induced cerebellar degeneration. This is confined to the vermis and spares the cerebellar hemispheres, explaining the upper extremities not being affected (normal finger-to-nose maneuver). *(Ref. 2, pp. 674–678)*

26. **E.** To demonstrate posterior fossa, sagittal MRI sections are most useful and would also show cerebellar-brainstem mass lesion if present. *(Ref. 2, p. 70)*

27. **A.** Unilateral Horner syndrome would cause anisocoria. Metabolic encephalopathy never causes pupillary abnormality unless it is due to medication which has a *direct* effect on the pupil. Pilocarpine eye drops have the same effect on both eyes. Diabetic ischemic oculomotor palsy *spares* the pupil. *(Ref. 2, pp. 191–195; Ref. 3, pp. 147–150)*

28. **A.** With pure CST lesion, weakness and Babinski sign are invariably present, as well as *hypotonia.* A finding of hypertonia (spasticity) usually develops in CST lesions but is not necessarily due directly to the CST lesion: It may be caused by vestibulospinal or reticulospinal tract involvement. *(Ref. 6, pp. 201–203)*

29. **D.** In aphasia, classification is based on verbal *comprehension, naming, spontaneous speech* and *repetition* abilities. Reading and writing may help assessment but are not essential to classify aphasia. *(Ref. 3, pp. 394–406)*

30. **E.** In assessing the optic disk, the presence of spontaneous venous pulsations (SVP) indicates that intracranial pressure is normal. Loss of SVP means that there is a *possibility* of increased intracranial pressure; however, some normal patients have *no* SVP. What is important is that if SVP are present, intracranial pressure is normal and LP can safely be performed. *(Ref. 2, pp. 184–187; Ref. 3, pp. 102–105)*

31. **A.** Cranial nuclei for the facial and abducens nerves are located in the dorsal pons, and CST travels through the ventral pons. Vascular ischemic pontine lesion would cause this clinical pattern. *(Ref. 2, pp. 276–277; Ref. 3, pp. 178–182)*

32. **E.** Gerstmann syndrome is due to lesion of the angular and supramarginal gyrus in the parietal lobe. All listed features involve utilization of hands–fingers and are part of this syndrome. *(Ref. 2, p. 426; Ref. 3, p. 405)*

33. **C.** In Anton's syndrome, the patient has cortical blindness with bilateral homonymous hemianopsia due to bilateral occipital lobe lesions. Anomia is the inability to name objects and is due to dominant-hemispheric lesions. Gait apraxia is due to bifrontal lesions. Amnesia is due to bitemporal lesions. Anosognosia is due to nondominant parietal lesions. *(Ref. 3, pp. 98, 517; Ref. 6, pp. 495–499)*

34. **C.** Oculo-palatal-pharyngeal myoclonus is rhythmical. It results from lesion within the dentate, red nucleus, and inferior olivary nucleus. Olives become enlarged. Patients may experience a clicking sound in the ear due to palatal myoclonus. *(Ref. 2, pp. 621–622; Ref. 3, pp. 265, 273)*

35. **C.** In "locked-in" syndrome, patients have severe motor impairment, with the only motor function being eye movements. Patients may communicate through these eye movements. This syndrome is due to a lesion in the *ventral* (bilateral) pons which spares eye movement centers and attention-consciousness centers in the *dorsal* pons. *(Ref. 2, p. 242; Ref. 3, pp. 457–458)*

36. **A.** Hemiballistic movements are due to neoplastic infectious-inflammatory or vascular (ischemic, hemorrhagic) lesion within the contralateral subthalamus. Sudden onset indicates that they are vascular in origin in this patient. *(Ref. 3, pp. 270–271; Ref. 6, pp. 466, 474)*

37. **A.** Wide-based, slapping gait is due to proprioceptive and spinal cord dysfunction due to neurosyphilis. With peroneal palsies, there is bilateral foot drop but gait is not usually broad-based. *(Ref. 2, pp. 146, 168, 469)*

38. **E.** In cerebellar lesions, all these findings are present. Ataxia of gait is most important, with impairment of performance of rapid alternating movements. Motor tone is floppy or hypotonic. *(Ref. 2, pp. 147–150; Ref. 3, pp. 287–290)*

39. **B.** With sciatic nerve injury, there is denervation of muscles supplied by both peroneal and posterior tibial muscles. This will mean there is no motor activity of the foot, leading to flail foot. *(Ref. 2, pp. 470–471; Ref. 3, p. 249)*

40. **A.** In traumatic head injury, these measures provide quick, reproducible, and semiquantitative clinical indications of the severity of brain injury. Initial score may provide a guide to prognosis. Based on patient score, clinical course can be followed by different examiners over time to determine if the patient is resolving or deteriorating in neurological status. *(Ref. 2, pp. 356–357)*

41. **E.** This type of injection *might* injure the sciatic nerve. This type of injury is avoided by injecting into the *upper-outer quadrant.* All listed muscles are innervated by the sciatic nerve. *(Ref. 2, pp. 470–471)*

42. **A.** Ischemic lesions in the left midbrain would cause dysfunction of the left oculomotor nerve and left CST to cause this clinical pattern. *(Ref. 2, pp. 276–277; Ref. 3, pp. 421–426)*

43. **B.** Corticospinal fibers are located in the capsule genu. Sensory fibers are located posterior and corticobulbar fibers are located in the anterior limb. *(Ref. 6, pp. 37–38)*

44. **A.** Alexia without agraphia (pure alexia) is due to dominant occipital lobe lesion. This also involves the splenium of the corpus callosum. With dominant occipital lobe lesion, right homonymous hemianopsia occurs. If the patient has writing difficulty (agraphia), the lesion is more likely located in the parietal region. *(Ref. 3, pp. 401, 405, 410;: Ref. 6, p. 498)*

45. **C**

46. **B**

47. **A**

48. **E**

49. **D**

45–49. In NPH, there is gait apraxia in which the legs have normal strength and coordination but cannot be utilized effectively for ambulation. There is usually associated dementia and incontinence, of which patient may not be cognizant. In ALS, there is motor impairment *only*, involving both upper and lower motor neurons. Reflexes are hyperactive and Babinski sign is positive because there are upper motor neuron signs. In syrinx, there is a central spinal cord cavity; therefore crossing lateral spinothalamic fibers are affected, causing "shawl-like" sensory disturbance. Also, anterior horn cells (which are located ventrally and medially) and emerging nerve roots may be affected, causing wasting and fasciculations of hands. If the patient has motor and sensory disturbances in both legs but with the arms spared, this indicates thoracic cord lesion. If the sacral (saddle) area is spared, this indicates that the process begins in the central portion of the cord and extends outward. If the saddle area is numb, this indicates extradural or intradural extramedullary cord lesion. "Crossed analgesia" refers to ipsilateral facial sensory anesthesia plus contralateral trunk and extremity anesthesia. This is indicative of brainstem lesion and is most characteristic of pontine localization, where the trigeminal fibers enter the brain stem. *(Ref. 2, pp. 168, 417–418, 604)*

50. **F**

51. **C**

52. **B**

53. **E**

54. **A**

55. **D**

50–55. Innervation of the peroneal nerve causes weakness of the foot dorsiflexor, resulting in "foot drop." The median nerve controls the thumb, so thumb flexion is weak. The ulnar nerve controls the fingers and use of the hand. With ulnar nerve weakness, there is "guttering" of fingers with weakness of finger adduction. The musculocutaneous nerve supplies the biceps muscle and if injured causes weak forearm flexion. *(Ref. 2, pp. 466–472; Ref. 6, pp. 342–343)*

56. B
57. A
58. C
59. E
60. D
61. G
62. F

56–62. Jaw jerk or masseter reflex is integrated through the mandibular trigeminal nerve in the pons. If hyperactive, this suggests brainstem lesion. Biceps reflex is mediated through C-5 and C-6 (predominantly C-6); triceps through C-7 and C-8 (predominantly C-7). Patellar or knee jerk is mediated through L-3 and L-4 (predominantly L-4); ankle jerk through S-1 and S-2 (predominantly S-1). Abdominal reflexes are superficial reflexes and with upper motor neuron lesions they are absent and *not* hyperactive (as is characteristic of *deep* tendon reflexes). Upper abdominal reflexes are mediated through T-8 and T-9; lower through T-10 to T-12. Cremasteric reflex is mediated by L-1 and L-2 and this is also a superficial reflex which is absent with upper motor neuron reflexes. In patients with suspected spinal cord or nerve root compression, it is important to know these reflex arcs. If the nerve root is compressed by an intervertebral disk, deep tendon reflexes will be diminished. *(Ref. 2, pp. 29–34; Ref. 6, pp. 220–230, 245–246)*

3

DIAGNOSTIC TESTS

True or False

1. _____ A skull radiogram will always show basilar skull fracture, and an isotope cisternogram is useful in assessing the source of CSF leakage causing otorrhea or rhinorrhea.

2. _____ An EEG is necessary to demonstrate the presence of spike discharges in patients suspected of having seizures; their presence always confirms a diagnosis of epilepsy.

3. _____ Nerve conduction velocities (NCV) are always slow in patients with polyneuropathy.

4. _____ An angiogram is required to confirm clinical suspicion of carotid artery occlusion.

5. _____ A myelogram is an important diagnostic study to show a herniated lumbar disk, but it is less sensitive than MRI and is associated with potentially dangerous side effects.

6. _____ CT and MRI visualize cerebral ventricles and subarachnoid spaces, and these are always enlarged in patients with Alzheimer's disease.

7. _____ Lumbar puncture with CSF analysis is usually necessary to diagnose bacterial, viral, and neoplastic meningitis; however, in some cases, it is justified to treat patients with suspected bacterial meningitis empirically, without first examining CSF.

8. _____ In patients with bacterial meningitis, the CSF shows lymphocytes and hypoglycorrhachia.

9. _____ The total amount of CSF is 150 cc, and it is located in the ventricles and subarachnoid spaces.

10. _____ The radionuclide isotope brain scan is the most sensitive study to demonstrate the integrity of the blood–brain barrier.

11. _____ The normal CSF protein content should not be more than 80 mg%, and the sugar content should be 66% of the blood sugar level.

12. _____ In patients with traumatic spinal tap and spontaneous subarachnoid hemorrhage, the CSF may appear xanthochromic, depending on the timing of LP.

13. _____ In multiple sclerosis, the CSF shows oligoclonal bands, the presence of myelin basic protein, and elevated gamma-globulin content.

14. _____ A positive India ink preparation indicates cryptococcal meningitis.

15. _____ MRI is superior to CT to demonstrate the full extent of tentorial, cerebellar, brainstem, and juxtasellar lesions.

16. _____ MRI is superior to CT for demonstrating intracranial calcifications.

17. _____ EEG can demonstrate abnormal electrical potentials in the thalamus and basal ganglia.

18. _____ An EEG should be perfomed in all patients who demonstrate unexplained changes in mental state.

19. _____ In patients with myasthenia gravis, repetitive nerve stimulation shows an *incremental* response.

20. _____ In a patient with mixed sensorimotor neuropathy of unexplained etiology, biopsy of both motor and sensory nerves should be performed.

21. _____ The presence of intracerebral and subarachnoid blood can always be detected by noncontrast CT.

22. _____ Conventional catheter angiography can delineate lenticulostriate arteriolar occlusion in patients with lacunar infarcts.

23. _____ Postcontrast CT or MRI is indicated in patients with suspected brain metastases.

24. _____ In patients with suspected parkinsonism and essential tremor, laboratory diagnostic tests are useful in establishing these diagnoses.

Multiple Choice

Choose the appropriate response.

25. _____ MRI is contraindicated in patients with:

    A. Cardiac pacemakers
    B. Artificial hips
    C. Prosthetic heart valves
    D. Eye implants
    E. All of the above

26. _____ Ammon horn sclerosis occurs in patients with this condition:

    A. Temporal lobe epilepsy
    B. Multiple sclerosis
    C. ALS
    D. Alzheimer's disease
    E. Parkinsonism

27. _____ Dystrophin is abnormal in patients with this condition:

    A. Duchenne dystrophy
    B. Myotonic dystrophy
    C. Charcot-Marie Tooth disease
    D. Neurofibromatosis
    E. Myasthenia gravis

28. _____ Acetylcholine receptor antibodies (AChR) are present in this condition:

    A. Polymyositis
    B. Myasthenia gravis
    C. Duchenne dystrophy
    D. Myotonic dystrophy
    E. Alzheimer's disease

29. _____ CSF findings which are consistent with cryptococcal meningitis include:

    A. Lymphocytic pleocytosis, low sugar, elevated protein
    B. Polymorphonuclear (PMN) pleocytosis, low sugar, elevated protein
    C. Lymphocytic pleocytosis, normal sugar, elevated protein
    D. Eosinophilic pleocytosis, normal sugar, elevated protein
    E. None of the above

30. _____ An important ancillary blood test in diagnosing psychogenic seizure is:

    A. Basal plasma cortisol
    B. Plasma growth hormone
    C. Serum prolactin
    D. Creatine kinase (CK)
    E. Serum calcium

31. _____ CT demonstrates brain structures due to:

    A. Differences in brain radiodensities
    B. Distribution of brain calcium content
    C. Differences in blood–brain barrier characteristics
    D. Distribution of brain water content
    E. None of the above

32. _____ Amyloid deposition in the brain occurs in patients with this condition:

    A. Alzheimer's disease
    B. Amyloid angiopathy
    C. Leukemia
    D. Multiple myeloma
    E. Plasmacytoma

33. _____ This is a human prion disease:

    A. Multiple sclerosis
    B. Jakob-Creutzfeldt disease
    C. Progressive multifocal leukoencephalopathy
    D. Parkinson's disease
    E. None of the above

34. _____ The most sensitive diagnostic study to detect early cerebral infarction is:

    A. Noncontrast CT
    B. Postcontrast CT
    C. Noncontrast MRI
    D. MRI with gadolinium
    E. Angiogram

RESPONSES AND EXPLANATIONS

1. **F.** A skull radiogram shows the brain and skull distribution of ionized calcium. They are *usually* useful for detecting bone discontinuities such as occur with a skull fracture; however, bones at the skull base are quite thin and a fracture line may be missed unless basal skull tomograms are also performed. With basilar skull fracture, the dura may be torn, causing CSF to leak; CSF pathways can be traced with an isotope cisternogram to show the site of CSF leakage. *(Ref. 2, pp. 43–48)*

2. **F.** EEG is helpful in confirming the presence of abnormal discharges in patients suspected of epilepsy; however, spikes may occur in patients *without* seizures or epilepsy. Treat patients, not EEG findings. If a clinical episode is *not* consistent with seizure, EEG findings alone should not be used to determine the need for antiepileptic medication. *(Ref. 1, pp. 67–72; Ref. 2, pp. 48–53)*

3. **F.** NCV are determined by the thickness and integrity of large myelinated fibers. In most *large* fiber neuropathies, NCV are slowed; however, with *small* fiber neuropathies, NCV may be normal. *(Ref. 1, pp. 77–81; Ref. 2, pp. 74–75; Ref. 5, pp. 157–176)*

4. **T.** Ultrasound is useful to demonstrate vascular stenosis. It is less useful to differentiate severe stenosis from occlusion, and this distinction requires angiography. Since this distinction has surgical implications (carotid endarterectomy is indicated for severe stenosis but not for occlusion), angiography is necessary to differentiate stenosis from occlusion. *(Ref. 1, p. 245; Ref. 2, pp. 56–57)*

5. **T.** Myelogram may show evidence that the spinal root or spinal cord is compressed, but this procedure requires LP and intrathecal injection of oil-based or water-soluble iodinated dye. MRI is more sensitive, as it shows actual changes (desiccation) of intervertebral disks as well as spinal root or spinal cord compression. *(Ref. 2, pp. 62–63)*

6. **F.** Both CT and MRI can demonstrate CSF in ventricles and subarachnoid spaces. Usually, these spaces are enlarged when the brain is shrunken in Alzheimer's disease; however, in some Alzheimer's patients, CSF spaces do *not* appear enlarged. Alternatively, in some patients with normal mental state, CSF spaces appear enlarged. *(Ref. 1, pp. 59–66; Ref. 2, pp. 63–71)*

7. **F.** CSF examination is mandatory to diagnose meningitis and to detect causal organisms by appropriate stains and cultures. In suspected meningitis, there is almost always time to perform LP prior to making treatment decisions. Meningitis can only be diagnosed by results of CSF analysis. If LP with CSF examination has *not* been performed, the patient cannot have *confirmed* diagnosis of meningitis. *(Ref. 1, pp. 93–96; Ref. 2, pp. 54–56)*

8. **F.** In bacterial meningitis, cellular response is predominantly polymorphonuclear leukocytes. Due to CSF white blood cell and CSF microorganism metabolic needs, CSF sugar is reduced (hypoglycorrhachia). In tuberculous and fungal meningitis, lymphocytes and low sugar are characteristic CSF formulas, and differentiation is established by appropriate stains, culture, and antigen results. *(Ref. 2, pp. 111–112, 537–550)*

9. **T.** Total CSF volume is 150 cc. This fluid is located in ventricles (50 cc) and cisternal spaces (100 cc). CSF is produced at rate of 0.3 cc/min, and CSF turns over approximately 6 times per day. It is produced by choroid plexus of the lateral third and fourth ventricles; reabsorption occurs through arachnoid granulations of the venous sinuses. *(Ref. 5, pp. 287–288)*

10. **F.** Radionuclide brain scan is positive when the blood–brain barrier is impaired; however, postcontrast CT and MRI are more sensitive studies to detect impaired blood–brain barrier. Isotope brain scan has less spatial resolution than CT or MRI; therefore it is not utilized when CT or MRI is available. *(Ref. 2, pp. 52–53)*

11. **F.** CSF protein should be less than 50 mg%. If it is elevated, this is a nonspecific marker of brain pathology. It is analogous to an "elevated blood ESR" in patients with suspected systemic illness. Elevated protein content indicates brain disease but provides no information as to specific type. CSF sugar content should be 66% of simultaneously drawn blood sugar and in all cases should be greater than 40 mg %. *(Ref. 2, pp. 542–543)*

12. **T.** The presence of CSF discoloration (xanthochromia) is dependent on the presence of red blood cells in CSF. If LP is traumatic, RBC enter CSF and unless CSF is rapidly centrifuged, CSF may appear xanthochromic. It takes several hours for xanthochromia to develop following subarachnoid hemorrhage; therefore, if LP is done immediately after spontaneous subarachnoid hemorrhage, CSF may not appear xanthochromic. *(Ref. 2, pp. 55–56)*

13. **T.** In multiple sclerosis, CSF shows abnormalities in 75–90% of cases. The elevated gamma-globulin content is diagnostic only when total CSF protein is normal. The presence of oligoclonal bands usually correlates with elevated gamma-globulin content. It is important to assess that CSF oligoclonal bands have not originated from the serum. The presence of myelin basic protein is quite specific for MS. *(Ref. 2, pp. 657–658)*

14. **T.** The use of India ink preparation demonstrates *encapsulated* yeast, and cryptococcus is the only such organism that invades CNS. The presence of elevated serum or CSF cryptococcal antigen is the most sensitive test for possible occurrence of cryptococcal meningitis. *(Ref. 2, p. 551)*

15. **T.** Because of alternate-plane reconstruction capability (coronal, sagittal), MRI is more sensitive and gives more precise anatomical detail than CT for lesions in all these locations. CT is usually done only in the transverse (axial) plane. *(Ref. 1, pp. 59–63; Ref. 2, pp. 70–71)*

16. **F.** CT is the most sensitive technique to demonstrate intracranial calcification. CT detects differences in *electron density* between intracranial tissues. Because of the nonmagnetic properties of calcium, it is not well visualized by MRI. *(Ref. 2, pp. 63–66)*

17. **F.** EEG demonstrates superficial cortical electrical potentials and therefore deeply situated potentials such as those originating from the thalamus and basal ganglia would not be easily detected. To detect such electrical potentials would require *depth* electrodes. *(Ref. 2, pp. 48–53)*

18. **T.** In patients with *unexplained* mental status changes, the possibility of behavioral or partial complex status epilepticus should be considered. To exclude this possibility, EEG is necessary. In most metabolic-toxic encephalopathies, EEG would be expected to show a *diffuse* slow wave pattern. *(Ref. 2, pp. 48–53; Ref. 4, pp. 80–81)*

19. **F.** In myasthenia gravis, repetitive nerve stimulation shows *decremental* muscle response due to abnormality of acetylcholine at the muscle receptor site. The diagnosis can be confirmed by positive response (increasing muscle strength) when the patient is injected with a cholinomimetic agent, edrophonium (Tensilon). Utilizing single-fiber EMG, the interval between evoked responses of muscle fibers in the same motor unit is measured. The interval may normally vary; this is called "jitter." In MG, jitter is *increased*. *(Ref. 2, pp. 528–529; Ref. 4, pp. 238–239)*

20. **F.** In certain neuropathies of undetermined etiology, biopsy of a pure *sensory* nerve, e.g., sural, greater auricular, might be warranted; however, following the biopsy, the area innervated by the nerve would be anesthetic. There would be no clinical indication to biopsy motor nerve, as this would result in weakness as muscles would become denervated. Sural nerve biopsy is warranted only when the etiology of neuropathy cannot be determined by noninvasive laboratory tests. *(Ref. 1, pp. 97–99; Ref. 2, pp. 76–77)*

21. **F.** CT is the most sensitive diagnostic test to detect intracerebral (parenchymal) blood. Blood appears as a hyperdense, nonenhancing lesion. CT is 100% sensitive for detecting intracerebral blood; for SAH detection, CT is less sensitive. The most sensitive test to detect SAH is LP with CSF analy-sis to detect the presence of RBC or xanthochromia. If CT is performed within 24 hr of SAH, blood is seen in 80% of cases; but within 48 hr, this positive rate falls off to 60%. Remember, when clinical diagnosis of SAH is most equivocal, CT is least likely to be positive and LP is most needed. *(Ref. 2, pp. 284–295)*

22. **F.** Angiography is the "gold standard" to detect *arterial* and *venous* intracranial vascular structures and abnormalities; however, *arterioles* are beyond the resolving capability of angiography and are not visualized. For example, angiography detects berry arterial aneurysm which causes SAH, but *not* Charcot-Bouchard arteriolar aneurysms which cause hypertensive intracerebral hemorrhages. *(Ref. 1, pp. 82–92; Ref. 2, pp. 59–62)*

23. **T.** In some cases, metastases appear as abnormal-density lesions on noncontrast CT or MRI; however, in some cases, use of intravenous contrast is necessary to detect metastases. In all patients with suspected brain metastases, postcontrast CT or MRI should be routinely performed. *(Ref. 2, p. 66; Ref. 5, pp. 323–340)*

24. **F.** The diagnosis of parkinsonism is established on a *clinical* basis and by clinical response to dopaminergic medication. If there are atypical clinical features, e.g., no resting tremor is present, consider CT or MRI to exclude hydrocephalus, multiple infarcts, or subdural hematoma. In progressive supranuclear palsy, which may simulate the clinical features of parkinsonism, CT or MRI may show midbrain abnormalities; whereas in PD, CT/MRI is usually normal. With SPECT and PET studies, abnormal basal ganglia metabolism may be detected, but this is not usually clinically useful. *(Ref. 4, p. 242)*

25. **A.** In patients with cardiac pacemakers and intracranial surgical metallic clips, e.g., those used for intracranial aneurysms, MRI should *not* be performed because of their magnetic properties. CT is a useful alternative procedure in such patients. *(Ref. 2, p. 72)*

26. **A.** In patients with partial complex seizures, atrophic pathological processes, including mesial temporal sclerosis, hamartomas, and cortical dysplasia, may occur. *(Ref. 4, pp. 168–169; Ref. 5, pp. 157–176)*

27. **A.** Dystrophin is a protein which is part of the cytoskeletal structure of muscle cells. It shares structural similarities with actinin and spectrin. Dystrophin is absent in muscles of patients with Duchenne dystrophy but *not* in other muscle dystrophy types. *(Ref. 2, pp. 506, 509–510)*

28. **E.** The pathogenesis of MG is due to the effects of autoantibodies to AChR. These antibodies are produced by the thymus gland. There is damage to muscle end plates. Most patients with generalized MG have these antibodies; however,

some patients with ocular MG alone have *no* antibodies. There is *no* correlation between antibody titer and severity of clinical symptoms of MG. *(Ref. 1, pp. 754–757; Ref. 2, pp. 529–530)*

29. **A.** In chronic meningitis of fungal or tuberculous origin, CSF shows *lymphocytic* pleocytosis. CSF sugar is reduced and protein is elevated. Cryptococcal antigen is positive and India ink preparation shows the encapsulated organism in cryptococcal meningitis. Eosinophils are seen with parasitic infection and polymorphonuclear cells are seen with bacterial meningitis. *(Ref. 2, pp. 537–550)*

30. **C.** Serum prolactin is elevated immediately following a partial complex seizure, but it will not be elevated after a psychogenic seizure. CK is likely to be elevated following a generalized seizure due to intense tonic-clonic muscle contraction, but it could also be elevated following an intense psychogenic seizure. The other hypothalamic pituitary hormones are not elevated following any type of seizure. Serum prolactin elevations occur very transiently and may return to normal within 30 min. *(Neurologic Clinics North America 12, pp. 31–40, 1994)*

31. **A.** CT is capable of differentiating brain structures due to differences in electron densities of the tissue. Despite the small differences in electron densities of gray matter, white matter, and CSF, they can be differentiated. If there is an impairment of the blood–brain barrier, postcontrast study will show abnormal tissue enhancement. *(Ref. 2, pp. 63–69)*

32. **A.** Amyloid is a protein seen in brain of patients with Alzheimer's disease. The major protein is a beta-A-4 peptide which is derived from amyloid precursor protein. The gene for amyloid is located on chromosome 21. Another protein seen in Alzheimer's disease is tau protein, which is a microtubule protein. *(Ref. 1, pp. 667–670)*

33. **B.** Other prion diseases include kuru, scrapie, Gerstmann-Straussler disease, and fatal familial insomnia. Prions are like viral particles in that they are transmissible, but they contain *no* nucleic acid. They contain protein and are infectious. *(Ref. 1, pp. 169–172, 682–683)*

34. **D.** CT does not show pathological changes related to cerebral infarction for many hours. MRI is more sensitive and may show abnormal water content within 4 hr; if contrast MRI is utilized, breakdown in the blood–brain barrier may be detected even earlier. Diffusion and perfusion weighted MRI may be even more sensitive and may detect abnormalities within 1–2 hr following ischemia. An angiogram may show vascular occlusion but does not show brain changes due to vascular occlusion. *(Ref. 1, pp. 243–245; Ref. 5, pp. 435–458)*

4

HEADACHE AND PAIN SYNDROMES

Multiple Choice

Choose the most appropriate response.

1. _____ During pregnancy, treatment of migraine may include:

   A. Ergot/caffeine
   B. DHE/Reglan
   C. Cafergot
   D. Amitriptyline
   E. Usually not necessary as migraine frequency and severity is reduced, and the above-listed drugs are contraindicated

2. _____ The following cranial structures are pain sensitive:

   A. Venous sinuses
   B. Meningeal arteries
   C. Head and neck muscles
   D. Large cranial arteries
   E. All of the above

3. _____ The following are characteristic of migraine without aura:

   A. Bilateral location of pain
   B. Thunderclap quality to pain onset
   C. Shock or jolt quality of pain
   D. Photopsia and microscopia are present
   E. Headache is associated with nasal congestion, lacrimation, and Horner syndrome

4. _____ The following is characteristic of migraine with aura:

   A. Fortification spectra
   B. Headache preceding motor weakness
   C. Headache preceding aphasia
   D. Amaurosis fugax and scintillating scotoma
   E. Headache precipitated by emotional stress

5. _____ The following is characteristic of "cluster-type" headache:

   A. Pupillary dilatation
   B. Relieved by sleep
   C. Long duration of pain episodes
   D. Prominent autonomic discharge during headache
   E. Diplopia during attack

6. _____ The following is characteristic of trigeminal neuralgia:

   A. Usually due to multiple sclerosis
   B. Episodes may be aborted by certain antiepileptic or antispasticity medications
   C. Sensory loss is detected on the face
   D. Weak masseter muscle function
   E. Bursts of pain last 30–60 min

7. _____ Effective treatment strategies for "status migrainous" include:

   A. Adequate fluid replacement
   B. DHE and Reglan
   C. Imitrex
   D. Phenothiazines
   E. All of the above

8. _____ A 30-year-old man develops "the first and worst headache of his life" after 5 min of weight lifting. The headache is throbbing in quality. It causes him to stop lifting. The headache disappears in 10 min. When he goes to the emergency department (ED), he is asymptomatic and the exam is entirely normal. What is the most likely diagnosis?

   A. Subarachnoid hemorrhage
   B. Bacterial meningitis
   C. Benign exertional headache
   D. Intracranial hypertension
   E. Hypertensive encephalopathy

9. _____ If you could perform *one* diagnostic study in this headache patient (question 8), which of the following would you choose?

   A. CT
   B. MRI
   C. Lumbar puncture with CSF examination
   D. Cerebral angiogram
   E. ESR

10. _____ This finding is characteristic of temporal arteritis:

   A. Throbbing headache
   B. Markedly elevated ESR

C. Tender temporomandibular joint
D. Active arthritis
E. Pulsatile, nontender temporal artery

11. _____ This neurotransmitter is involved in migraine:

A. Dopamine
B. Acetylcholine
C. Serotonin
D. GABA
E. Norepinephrine

12. _____ If a patient has thunderclap headache and CT scan shows blood in the left sylvian fissure, the next diagnostic study would be:

A. EEG
B. MRI
C. LP
D. Left carotid angiogram
E. Four-vessel cerebral angiogram

13. _____ Intermittent Horner syndrome may be seen in this headache disorder:

A. Migraine with aura
B. Migraine without aura
C. Temporal arteritis
D. Benign intracranial hypertension
E. Cluster

14. _____ This characteristic would be unusual in migraine patients:

A. Vicelike pain
B. Associated nausea
C. Initial unilateral headache
D. Visual prodrome to headache
E. Photophobia

15. _____ Migraine symptoms are most likely due to:

A. Vasoconstriction
B. Epileptiform discharges
C. Cerebral edema
D. Decreased cerebral metabolism due to spreading cortical depression
E. Vasodilatation

16. _____ These drugs are effective in acute migraine management:

A. Isometheptene, dichloralphenazone
B. Ergotamine
C. Caffeine
D. Imitrex
E. All of the above

17. _____ The major side effect of dihydroergotamine (DHE) in migraine management is:

A. Vasoconstriction
B. Seizures
C. Nausea
D. Altered mental state
E. Visual loss

18. _____ Characteristic features of major causalgia are:

A. Burning dysesthetic symptoms
B. Associated dystrophic nail changes
C. Limb temperature changes
D. Relief with nerve block
E. All of the above

19. _____ Complications of ruptured berry aneurysm include:

A. Recurrence of bleeding
B. Vasospasm
C. Hyponatremia
D. Hydrocephalus
E. All of the above

20. _____ Complications of pseudotumor cerebri include:

A. Visual loss
B. Hydrocephalus
C. Seizures
D. Gait apraxia
E. Oculomotor nerve paresis

21. _____ The following is true of trigeminal neuralgia:

A. Pain may extend to the ear
B. Lancinating bursts of pain last seconds
C. Ophthalmic division of trigeminal nerve is affected most frequently
D. Corneal reflex is diminished
E. Pain is exacerbated by wine or cheese ingestion

22. _____ Paroxysmal burst of pain lasting seconds, localized to tongue, tonsils, or auditory meatus, is defined as:

A. Postherpetic neuralgia
B. Trigeminal neuralgia
C. Cluster headache
D. Glossopharyngeal neuralgia
E. Sphenoid sinusitis

23. _____ Potential side effects of beta-receptor antagonists used for migraine treatment may include:

A. Bradycardia
B. Weight gain
C. Heart failure
D. Asthma exacerbation
E. All of the above

24. _____ Medications utilized for migraine prophylaxis are:

A. Dihydroergotamine
B. Indomethacin
C. Acetazolamide
D. Calcium channel blockers
E. Sumatriptan

True or False

From the clinical history, answer true or false.

S.B. is a 25-year-old woman who comes to see you for evaluation of a headache that she says has lasted "10 years." She has had a headache upon awakening every day for the last 2 years. It is bifrontal or occipital, usually described as "pressure pain," and, when severe, can cause nausea. Glare bothers her when driving. She has chronic tiredness, but cannot sleep well. She works as a secretary. She used to exercise, but had to quit playing tennis and jogging, as these activities exacerbated her headache.

   She has had head CT, which is normal. She utilized Inderal, but it was not effective and made her feel like a "zombie." Elavil was not helpful. At present, she self-medicates herself with Goodies Powders, up to 4 packets per day, Excedrin PM, 2 q.h.s., Advil on occasion, Sudafed almost daily. She uses oral contraceptive pills (OCP), and she smokes 1 pack per day. She drinks caffeine, 2 cups of coffee every morning and 4 diet cokes per day, because this "helps my headache."

25. _____ S.B. has had adequate pharmacotherapy for her chronic headache, including preventative and abortive medications.

26. _____ S.B. should not exercise until she undergoes angiogram to rule out AVM or aneurysm.

27. _____ S.B. is addicted to analgesics.

28. _____ Birth control pills are contraindicated in SB's condition.

Multiple Choice

From the clinical history, choose the appropriate response.

A 19-year-old college student develops scintillating scotoma following by left throbbing headache associated with vomiting. This recurs four times in one semester, always immediately after a major course examination. Both parents have migraine. Neurological examination is normal.

29. _____ Which diagnostic test should be performed?

A. CT
B. LP

C. EEG
D. Angiogram
E. None of the above

30. _____ The most appropriate therapy would include:

A. Prophylactic beta-blocking agent
B. Prophylactic calcium channel blocker
C. Abortive agent when visual symptoms begin
D. Abortive agent taken when headache begins
E. Biofeedback

31. _____ The following is true of this patient:

A. Stress precipitates headache
B. Patient has high risk of stroke
C. Patient has high risk of epilepsy
D. Psychotherapy is warranted to reduce stress
E. None of the above

A 28-year-old medical student develops severe bifrontal headache after weight lifting. The patient's headache recedes 5 min after he stops this activity. Exam in the ED of the local hospital is normal.

32. _____ Which is the most likely diagnosis?

A. Acute bacterial meningitis
B. Subarachnoid hemorrhage
C. Benign exertional headache
D. Cluster headache
E. Pseudotumor cerebri

33. _____ What diagnostic tests should be performed?

A. LP
B. CT
C. MRI
D. Angiogram
E. None of the above

34. _____ Which medication should be utilized?

A. Indomethacin
B. Dexamethasone
C. Mannitol
D. Intubation with hyperventilation
E. Diamox

True or False

M.R. develops symptoms characteristic of migraine with aura. He has had 5 attacks in 5 years, and headaches respond to Imitrex. His neurological examination is normal. He has positive family history for migraine and experienced motion sickness as a child. He goes to his family physician, who believes that diagnostic studies should be performed to confirm the diagnosis of migraine.

Based on the above case history, answer true or false.

35. _____ Diagnostic studies can confirm diagnosis of migraine.

36. _____ CT or MRI with contrast should be performed to exclude "brain lesion."

37. _____ The finding of "venous angioma" by CT or MRI would change management.

38. _____ CT or MRI should be performed as possible protection against subsequent malpractice litigation.

39. _____ Vascular imaging procedure should be done, since migraine patients have increased incidence of stroke.

40. _____ EEG should be performed, since migraine patients have increased incidence of epilepsy.

Multiple Choice

A 45-year-old man develops bifrontal throbbing headaches which persist for 2 hr and then disappear, only to return 6 hr later. He has no prior headache history. On two occasions, he has vomited and had transient visual obscurations. After 6 days of headache, he goes to the ED and is given Demerol and Vistaril for migraine. The headache disappears for 2 days but then recurs. Funduscopy shows no spontaneous venous pulsations; neurological examination is otherwise normal.

Based on the above case history, choose the appropriate response.

41. _____ The most likely diagnosis would be:

    A. Migraine with aura
    B. Migraine without aura
    C. Cluster
    D. Sphenoid sinusitis
    E. None of the above

42. _____ When the headache recurs, the next management step should be:

    A. Imitrex therapeutic trial
    B. DHE therapeutic trial
    C. CT
    D. LP
    E. ESR

43. _____ Based on clinical information, the following abnormality might be seen on CT:

    A. Colloid cyst without hydrocephalus
    B. Colloid cyst with hydrocephalus
    C. Pituitary adenoma
    D. Craniopharyngioma
    E. All of the above

44. _____ The mechanism of headache due to intracranial neoplasm is:

    A. Traction of pain-sensitive structure
    B. Cerebral edema
    C. Hydrocephalus
    D. Intracranial hypertension
    E. All of the above

A 42-year-old man develops right-frontal aching-quality headache. He reports paresthesias in the eyebrow region and horizontal diplopia. He has fever but feels well otherwise. He has *no* prior history of headache. The headache worsens over 1 week, it awakens the patient from sleep, and it does not respond to conventional analgesics.

45. _____ Diagnostic possibilities include:

    A. Sinusitis
    B. Migraine with aura
    C. Migraine without aura
    D. Cluster
    E. Tension headache

46. _____ Exam shows reduced pinprick over the ophthalmic branch of the trigeminal nerve, ptosis, lateral and medial recti, and weakness on the right side. Diagnostic possibilities include:

    A. Sphenoid sinusitis
    B. Pituitary adenoma
    C. Meningitis
    D. Subarachnoid hemorrhage
    E. None of the above

47. _____ The most important diagnostic study would be:

    A. Skull radiogram
    B. LP
    C. CT
    D. ESR
    E. None of the above

48. _____ The only intracranially located sinus is the:

    A. Sphenoid
    B. Maxillary
    C. Frontal
    D. Ethmoid
    E. None of the above

A 35-year-old woman has had "migraine" since her college years. She has left-sided visual disturbances followed by right-sided throbbing headaches associated with vomiting. These occur once every 6 months and resolve completely with Cafergot. In addition, she has headaches without visual disturbances 3 times per week, for which she takes Fiorinal with aspirin. In the last 6 months, she has had chronic daily headaches which are bitemporal, aching pain and interfere with sleep. They do not respond to Cafergot and she is taking 20 Fiorinal tablets per day. Neurological examination is completely normal.

49. _____ The most likely diagnosis of the new headache would be:

A. Cluster
B. Migraine without aura
C. Chronic daily headache due to transformed migraine
D. Intracranial neoplasm
E. Chronic meningitis

50. _____ The most appropriate diagnostic test would be:

A. CT
B. MRI
C. LP
D. ESR
E. None of the above

The Fiorinal is stopped because the patient develops severe abdominal pain. Two days later, she has a generalized seizure.

51. _____ The most likely mechanism of the seizure is:

A. Brain neoplasm
B. Meningitis
C. Subarachnoid hemorrhage
D. Barbiturate withdrawal
E. None of the above

A 45- year-old man has a 10-year history of episodes of lancinating sharp right eye pain associated with nasal congestion and lacrimation. Each episode lasts 50 min and awakens the patient from sleep. He has episodes which last 2 weeks and then stop spontaneously. Over the last year, headache has been occurring more frequently such that he has headache every 3 days. Each headache lasts 10 min and occurs 5 times each day and has jabbing and throbbing quality. Neurological exam is normal.

52. _____ The most likely diagnosis for the initial headache is:

A. Migraine without aura
B. Cluster
C. Tension
D. All of the above
E. None of the above

53. _____ The most effective acute abortive treatment would be:

A. Nasal oxygen
B. Fiorinal
C. Oral cafergot
D. Narcotics
E. Beta-adrenergic agents

54. _____ The most likely diagnosis for the most recent headache is:

A. Cluster
B. Migraine without aura
C. Chronic paroxysmal hemicrania
D. Tension
E. None of the above

55. _____ Effective treatment for the new headache would be:

A. Indomethacin
B. Elavil
C. Prednisone
D. Calcium channel blockers
E. All of the above

56. _____ Because the headache pattern has changed, this diagnostic study should be considered:

A. Skull radiogram
B. CT
C. MRI
D. LP
E. None of the above

TP is a 28-year-old woman evaluated for "migraine." She has positive family history for migraine and had motion sickness as a child. In addition, she has episodes of chest pain, palpitations, and intense fear. Her headache begins with fortification spectrum followed 20 min later by right-temporal throbbing headache and vomiting. She has 2 attacks per week. In addition, her appetite is poor, she awakens 3 times per night, and she feels "blue." Neurological examination is normal.

57. _____ Which neurodiagnostic study should be performed?

A. CT
B. MRI
C. EEG
D. LP
E. None of the above

58. _____ Which of the following is associated with migraine as a comorbid condition?

A. Affective disorder
B. Mitral valve prolapse
C. Peptic ulcer disease
D. Epilepsy
E. All of the above

59. _____ During acute attack, which agent should be initially utilized?

    A. Cafergot
    B. Imitrex
    C. Dihydroergotamine
    D. Calcium channel blocker
    E. Phenothiazine (Thorazine)

60. _____ If the episode does not resolve with initial therapy, which management strategy should be considered?

    A. Intravenous fluids
    B. Imitrex
    C. Dihydroergotamine
    D. Reglan
    E. All of the above

61. _____ Following control of the acute attack, which drug would be contraindicated as prophylactic treatment?

    A. Elavil
    B. Inderal
    C. Verapamil
    D. Depakote
    E. Prozac

62. _____ If the patient developed episodes in which she felt dizzy, light-headed, experienced visual gray-out and then lost consciousness, falling limply to the ground, the most likely diagnosis would be:

    A. Migraine stroke
    B. Syncope
    C. Seizure
    D. Drug-induced effect
    E. None of the above

63. _____ The following is true of myofascial pain syndromes:

    A. Trigger points are present
    B. Fatigue is commonly reported
    C. Sleep disturbances are common
    D. Neurological exam is normal
    E. All of the above

RESPONSES AND EXPLANATIONS

1. **E.** Acetaminophen and meperidine can be recommended for use during pregnancy; however, *any* drug presents potential risk during pregnancy. Aspirin may prolong labor, cause blood loss during pregnancy, and increase risk of stillbirth. Ergot may cause placental damage due to vasoconstrictive effect. Fortunately, migraine tends to remit during pregnancy. New-onset headache during pregnancy should be evaluated carefully for potential vascular or structural lesion. *(Ref. 1, p. 965; Ref. 2, p. 706)*

2. **E.** Pain-sensitive structures include:

   a. Proximal portion of large extra- and intracranial arteries
   b. Large veins and venous sinuses
   c. Meninges
   d. Upper cervical nerve roots
   e. Cranial nerves V, IX, and X

   Brain parenchyma is pain-insensitive, as are ventricles and choroid plexus. Electrode stimulation of the periaqueductal gray (PAG) region and somatosensory thalamus may cause headache. The descending analgesic system includes the mid-brain PAG, medial medullary raphe nucleus, reticular formation, and dorsal horn neurons of the spinal cord. *(Ref. 1, pp. 43–44)*

3. **C.** Head shocks or jolts are quite characteristic of migraine. Pain begins as *unilateral* headache but later becomes bilateral. Thunderclap pattern or sudden increase to maximal pain severity suggests subarachnoid hemorrhage. Visual phenomena suggest migraine *with* aura, and *autonomic* features suggest *cluster*. *(Ref. 1, pp. 42–45)*

4. **A.** Fortification spectra are the most characteristic visual disturbance of migraine. These consist of C-shaped serrated zig-zag arcs followed by scotoma (area of blindness). Visual disturbance recedes before headache develops. When headache *precedes* neurological disturbance, consider nonmigraine disorders. Amaurosis fugax is visual loss in one eye only and suggests severe carotid stenosis. Emotional stress may precipitate migraine. Migraine usually develops not at peak stress but during a period of relaxation ("let-down"). This is contrasted with tension headache, which correlates directly with severity of emotional stress. *(Archives of Neurology 36, p. 784, 1979; Ref. 5, pp. 111–114)*

5. **D.** In cluster, patients *awaken* with severe short-lived headache. This is associated with autonomic dysfunction and Horner syndrome. The presence of headache with diplopia should suggest ruptured carotid aneurysm with oculomotor nerve dysfunction (ptosis, pupillary dilation, and extraocular muscle dysfunction). *(Neurologic Clinics of North America 75, pp. 579–591, 1991; Ref. 2, pp. 99–100)*

6. **B.** Trigeminal neuralgia develops due to demyelination of the trigeminal nerve (sensory portion). This could be due to MS plaque, neoplasm in the cerebello-pontine angle, or vascular lesion compressing the trigeminal nerve. In *most* cases of trigeminal neuralgia, *no* etiology is found and neurological examination is normal. Bursts of "electrical shock" pain usually last less than 30 sec and are confined to one division of the trigeminal nerve (mandibular is most common). Prior to diagnosis being established, dental origin for pain is considered, and many patients undergo unnecessary tooth extractions. Treatment includes carbamazepine, phenytoin, or baclofen. Surgical rhizotomy may be needed if medical therapy is not effective. There is a theory that the pain is due to compression of the trigeminal nerve by abnormal blood vessels, and if this is the case, microvascular decompression would be warranted. *(Ref. 2, pp. 114–116)*

7. **E.** As a result of vomiting, dehydration may be a significant problem. This should be corrected, and pain is frequently relieved by rehydration only. Subcutaneous Imitrex is effective, but injection may need to be repeated due to pain recurrence. Parenterally administered phenothiazines may be effective but may cause postural hypotension. Dihydroergotamine (DHE) and antiemetic (metoclopramide) Reglan are usually effective in refractory migraine. *(New England Journal of Medicine 329, pp. 1476–1482, 1993; Ref. 2, pp. 101–103)*

8. **C.** Sudden "thunderclap" headache suggests subarachnoid hemorrhage (SAH). Because the headache lasts only 10 min and then resolves, this suggests effort migraine, especially since the patient has no meningeal signs. It would be unlikely for pain of SAH to resolve rapidly. Lack of fever excludes meningitis; normal blood pressure excludes hypertensive encephalopathy; lack of papilledema excludes intracranial hypertension. *(Lancet 2, pp. 1247–1248, 1986)*

9. **C.** The major risk in this patient is SAH. Lumbar puncture with CSF analysis looking for red blood cells and blood breakdown products (xanthochromia) is most sensitive study. CT and MRI are not as sensitive as LP to detect SAH. Angiogram would only be warranted if CSF confirms diagnosis of SAH. *(Ref. 2 pp. 55–56)*

10. **B.** Headache is more commonly aching than throbbing. Jaw pain may occur with chewing, but TMJ tenderness is not usually present. The patient complains of joint pain and stiffness (polymyalgia rheumatica), but no active arthritis *is* found. The temporal artery is nonpulsative and frequently tender. ESR is usually markedly elevated. *(American Journal of Medicine 67, pp. 839–845, 1972; Ref. 2, pp. 112–113)*

11. **C.** It is believed that there is unstable *serotonin* neurotransmission in migraine, with increased raphe neuronal firing rates. During acute migraine attack, platelet serotonin levels fall and urinary serotonin increases. Serotonin transmission abnormalities in the gastrointestinal system explain prominent GI symptoms, and affective-mood disturbances are also due to unstable CNS serotonin changes. Drugs that treat migraine affect serotonin receptors. *(Ref. 4, p. 44)*

12. **E.** The term *thunderclap headache* implies that headache is sudden and severe. This pattern should alert the physician to the possibility of SAH. Although LP with CSF exam is the most definitive diagnostic study for SAH, CT was done and showed findings characteristic of ruptured middle cerebral artery aneurysm. Since 20% of aneurysms are multiple, a four-vessel angiogram is needed to study the entire cerebral circulation; whereas a left carotid angiogram would likely show the causal aneurysm only and not screen for the possibility of *multiple* aneurysms. *(Lancet 2, pp. 1247–1248, 1986; Postgraduate Medicine 86, pp. 93–100, 1989)*

13. **E.** Intermittent Horner syndrome is most likely to occur with cluster, due to distention of the internal carotid artery wall as the sympathetic fibers travel within the carotid artery. Horner syndrome is partial, with ptosis and miosis but no anhidrosis. Other autonomic signs are present (perspiration, tachycardia, bradycardia, lacrimation), which suggests autonomic instability. *(Medical Clinics of North America 75, pp. 579–591, 1986)*

14. **A.** Headache quality may be dull, aching, or pulsatile. The presence of jabbing, jolting, or shocklike pain may also occur. A band or vicelike pain is more characteristic of tension headache. Initially the headache is unilateral; it may then become bilateral. *(Ref. 2, pp. 92–94)*

15. **D.** Studies of migraine have focused on vascular factors indicating that vasoconstrictive drugs reduce the amplitude of pulsation in the superficial temporal artery but that this does not always reduce headache. It is believed that extracranial vasodilation is the cause of headache and intracranial vasoconstriction is the cause of neurological symptoms. Currently, the concept that "spreading cortical depression," which is a primary *neural* (not vascular) event, is the major migraine mechanism. This cortical depression leads to hypometabolic state and hypoperfusion. The role of unstable serotonergic neurotransmission in this cortical depression in migraine is being explored. *(Neurology 43 [suppl. 3], p. 51, 1993; Journal of Neurophysiology 7, pp. 359–390, 1941; Ref. 5, pp. 83–105)*

16. **E.** All listed agents are effective in treating migraine. Isometheptene in combination with acetaminophen and dichloralphenazone (Midrin) as well as caffeine are effective, possibly due to vasoconstrictive effect, despite the debate as to whether vascular factors are primary or secondary. These medications also affect serotonin receptors. Ergotamine is most effective when used parenterally and is less effective orally. Caffeine may enhance the effect of ergotamine. Imitrex is most effective and is a serotonin receptor agonist. *(Ref. 4, pp. 18–19)*

17. **C.** DHE is a weak vasoconstrictive agent compared to other ergot medications. However, in rare instances, idiosyncratic reactions may cause severe coronary or peripheral vascular spasm. Due to significant *emetic* complications, prochlorperazine or metoclopramide are administered before DHE. Avoid DHE in pregnancy. *(New England Journal of Medicine 329, pp. 1476–1491, 1993; Ref. 2, pp. 101–102)*

18. **E.** In patients with sympathetically mediated pain (reflex sympathetic dystrophy, major causalgia), pain characteristically is *burning* in quality, and pain occurs in response to stimulus, e.g., light touch that is not usually painful (allodynia). There are signs to indicate autonomic dysfunction (edema, erythema, cold limb, loss of hair and nail pattern), muscle wasting, and bone atrophy in the involved limb. Selective sympathetic nerve block abolishes pain temporarily, and sympathectomy may provide permanent relief. *(Ref. 1, pp. 486–488; Ref. 2, pp. 173–174)*

19. **E.** Congenital berry arterial aneurysm may rupture into subarachnoid spaces. Blood clots may occlude arachnoid granulations in basal cisterns, resulting in *hydrocephalus*. Blood may release neurotransmitters, resulting in vasospasm. SAH may lead to cerebral salt wasting and hyponatremia. The major risk of berry aneurysm is that there are multiple aneurysmal bleeding points and *rebleeding* will occur. *(Ref. 2, pp. 290–296)*

20. **A.** In patients with pseudotumor cerebri (idiopathic intracranial hypertension), the major threat is visual acuity loss. Ventricles are never enlarged and transtentorial (uncal) herniation never occurs. Gait apraxia occurs with normal-pressure hydrocephalus. *(Ref. 2, p. 110)*

21. **B.** In this disorder, pain occurs in bursts lasting seconds but there may be constant aching pain superimposed upon the brief pain bursts. Pain is confined to trigeminal nerve distribution (the ear is *beyond*) and usually involves the mouth (mandibular branch). Chewing or brushing teeth exacerbates pain. *(Ref. 2, pp. 114–115)*

22. **D.** Glossopharyngeal neuralgia is less common than trigeminal neuralgia. The pain characteristics are similar but the location is different. Swallowing, especially of cold liquids, triggers this pain. Syncope may occur in some patients due to vagal mediated bradycardia. Postherpetic neuralgia remains confined to the trigeminal nerve distribution, usually the ophthalmic division. *(Ref. 2, p. 114)*

23. **E.** Bradycardia, weight gain, and sluggish feeling (depression) are common side effects of beta-blocking adrenergic medications. Exacerbation of congestive heart failure or asthma

may occur. The mechanism of action in migraine may be independent of beta-receptor blockade but may involve an effect on serotonin transmission. *(Ref. 2, pp. 104–105)*

24. **D.** Migraine treatment may be abortive or prophylactic. Drugs that affect the serotonergic brainstem raphe system—ergot alkaloids, cyproheptadine, methysergide, calcium channel blockers, beta-blockers—are effective in prophylaxis of migraine; whereas other drugs are effective in aborting an acute attack. *(Ref. 2, pp. 101–105)*

25. **F**
26. **F**
27. **T**
28. **T**

25–28. Several other prophylactic medications also influence serotonin neurotransmission and may be utilized. These drugs include methysergide (Sansert), gamma-aminobutyric acid enhancers (Valproic acid), calcium channel blockers, and monamine oxidase (MAO) inhibitors. The patient has chronic daily headaches and it is most unlikely that there is an underlying structural or vascular lesion. Certainly, there could be *incidental* comorbid unsuspected intracranial lesions, but that is unlikely to be the *cause* of the headaches. This patient is dependent on analgesics, and analgesic-related headaches are occurring. Withdrawal from analgesics may allow development of a headache-free period, but caffeine, butalbital, or diazepam may cause withdrawal symptoms. Oral contraceptives are not contraindicated unless the patient has a family history of stroke, is hypertensive, older than 35, or smokes cigarettes. Low-estrogen-content oral contraceptives should be utilized. Obviously, if the headaches worsen when using OCP, they should be stopped and the patient switched to another type of OCP or utilize an alternative birth-control technique. *(Ref. 2, pp. 101–105)*

29. **E**
30. **E**
31. **E**

29–31. This is a classic example of migraine with aura. With positive family history, onset in the "let-down" phase after stress is over, and normal neurological exam, the yield from diagnostic studies would be low. For migraine attacks occurring less often than once per month, prophylactic therapy would not be warranted. If biofeedback can *abort* the attack, this would be ideal. If not, utilize medication as soon as visual symptoms begin. There is no evidence that ergot medication is dangerous or worsens visual symptoms. Emotional factors play a role in migraine, with a high incidence of psychiatric comorbid conditions (panic, anxiety, depression, mania), but migraine frequently occurs in the let-down period after the maximal period of stress has passed. In some unusual migraine patients, stroke or epilepsy may develop. *(Ref. 2, pp. 97–98)*

32. **C**
33. **E**
34. **A**

32–34. This is most likely "effort" migraine or "benign exertional headache." The short duration of the headache, receding after exercise stops, and normal neurological examination are *not* consistent with SAH. Cluster headache awakens the patient; meningitis is associated with fever and stiff neck; pseudotumor patients have papilledema. Headache similar to exertional migraine occurs in patients with cough due to respiratory infections. I would perform no diagnostic study in this case, but to be *certain* there is no SAH, LP would be the definitive study. Exertional headache is *indomethacin* responsive; however, the mechanism of medication effect is not established. The other listed medications reduce intracranial hypertension, which is not present in this case. *(Headache 28, p. 675, 1988; Journal of Neurology, Neurosurgery, and Psychiatry 57, pp. 134–150, 1994)*

35. **F**
36. **F**
37. **F**
38. **F**
39. **F**
40. **F**

35–40. Migraine is the clinical diagnosis and neurodiagnostic studies will be negative. CT/MRI is unnecessary in the classic migraine patient. A venous angioma is an incidental finding. Surgery is unnecessary, and its presence does not change migraine management. If the physician is concerned about being held culpable for incidental comorbid brain lesions, then CT/MRI should be performed on *all* headache patients. This is unnecessary! If there are atypical features, e.g., headache precedes visual symptoms, perform CT/MRI. Angiography is not necessary in migraine unless there are unusual features which suggest "migraine stroke," e.g., persistence of visual or other neurological features. Many patients with migraine have EEG abnormalities, but EEG is indicated only if the patient has an observed seizure. Remember, *syncope* is common in migraine, due to autonomic instability. Syncope should be readily differentiated from seizures. *(Ref. 2, pp. 85–95; Ref. 4, pp. 16–20)*

41. **E**
42. **C**
43. **B**
44. **E**

41–44. With no prior headache history and transient visual obscurations, the possibility of intracranial hypertension must be considered. When headache is intractable, CT should be performed to exclude intracranial pathology, as this headache history is worrisome. A midline tumor which is obstructing CSF pathways should be considered, especially since funduscopic exam shows early signs of papilledema with loss of spontaneous venous pulsations. A colloid cyst with hydrocephalus would be most likely to cause intracranial hypertension only; pituitary adenoma or craniopharyngioma would cause visual chiasmal signs, e.g., bitemporal hemianopsia. All listed mechanisms may cause headache in patients with brain masses. *(Ref. 2, pp. 108–111)*

45. **A**
46. **A**
47. **C**
48. **A**

45–48. Headache caused by sinus infection may awaken the patient from sleep. As the patient is out of bed, sinus drainage is enhanced and the headache disappears. The presence of ophthalmic branch of trigeminal nerve sensory disturbance with the finding of diplopia suggests the possibility of cavernous sinus involvement. A special form of migraine called *ophthalmoplegic migraine* could simulate this clinical pattern; however, this is a diagnosis of exclusion, after all neuroimaging studies including angiography are negative. With *sphenoid sinusitis,* extension to the cavernous sinus may occur, causing the listed neurological signs. CT would be the best study to show sphenoid and cavernous sinus abnormality. Since the sphenoid sinus is the only *intracranial* sinus, infection can cause neural involvement. Remember, the presence of fever suggests infection, and fever is *not* seen with migraine. LP may be necessary to exclude meningitis. *(New England Journal of Medicine 319, pp. 1149–1154, 1983; Ref. 2, pp. 106–107)*

49. **C**
50. **E**
51. **D**
52. **B**

49–52. The patient initially had migraine with aura. This *transformed* to chronic daily headache. The reason for the transformation is probably analgesic dependence. Whenever headache changes characteristics, diagnostic studies should be considered; however, this pattern is so characteristic that diagnostic studies are not warranted, especially since neurological examination is normal. Fiorinal contains butalbital and the seizure is barbiturate withdrawal seizure rather than a sign of intracranial lesion. Withdrawal seizure is generalized. If the seizure were focal, the possibility of underlying structural lesion would be considered. *(Neurology 47, pp. 871–875, 1996)*

53. **A**
54. **C**
55. **A**
56. **E**

53–56. Cluster develops suddenly, without warning, awakens the patient from sleep, and is usually located around the eye or temple region. The headache lasts 30–120 min and occurs in clusters or cycles. There are associated autonomic signs including lacrimation, conjunctival injection, and Horner syndrome. During acute attack, inhalation of 100% oxygen via nasal mask at a flow rate of 8–10 L/min for 10 min is the most effective therapy. Prophylactic therapy includes corticosteroids, lithium, ergotamine, or calcium-channel blockers. The new headache is more constant but has bursts of pain. This suggests *hemicrania continua,* which is an indomethacin-responsive headache. I would suggest using this medication prior to performing any diagnostic studies. *(Ref. 2, pp. 99–100)*

57. **E**
58. **E**
59. **A**
60. **B**
61. **B**
62. **B**

57–62. This young woman has positive family history for migraine and experienced motion sickness as a child. The latter is very common in migraine patients. In addition, cardiac symptoms suggest mitral valve prolapse and behavioral symptoms suggest affective disorder, both of which are comorbid disorders with migraine. Other comorbid conditions for migraine include peptic ulcer disease, colitis, epilepsy, and bipolar disorder. Because clinical features are so characteristic of migraine with aura, no neurodiagnostic studies are needed. During *early* migraine phase, utilize Cafergot initially. If Cafergot is not effective, utilize Imitrex. Fluid replacement may be warranted if the patient has had vomiting and appears dehydrated. Be careful in the choice of prophylactic agents for migraine. Inderal would be a good choice for a patient with mitral valve prolapse but not if the patient has depressive symptoms. In patients with depression, Elavil would be a better choice. *(Seminars in Neurology 11, pp. 118–127, 1991)*

63. **E.** There is similarity between this and fibromyalgia and chronic fatigue syndrome. Sleep disturbances are common and appear to exacerbate the musculoskeletal disorder. Treatment with physical therapy, tricyclic antidepressants, and nonsteroidal antiinflammatory drugs is effective. *(Ref. 2, pp. 718–719)*

5

SPINAL CORD DISEASE; NECK AND BACK PAIN

Multiple Choice

Choose the most appropriate response.

1. _____ A 56-year-old man is involved in a motor vehicle accident during which his head hits the steering wheel. Following the accident, he reports neck pain and stiffness on flexion, extension, and lateral neck rotation. Neurological exam is normal. Likely diagnostic possibilities include:

   A. Subarachnoid hemorrhage (SAH)
   B. Acute cervical strain
   C. Cervical spondylosis
   D. Cervical myelopathy
   E. Cervical radiculopathy

2. _____ Clinical findings due to S-1 radiculopathy include:

   A. Absent ankle (Achilles) reflex
   B. Weakness of foot dorsiflexion
   C. Neurogenic bladder
   D. Positive unilateral Babinski sign
   E. All of the above

3. _____ A herniated T-8 thoracic disk may cause which of these findings:

   A. Paraparesis
   B. Autonomic bladder
   C. Bilateral Babinski signs
   D. Absent abdominal reflexes
   E. All of the above

4. _____ Clinical features of carpal tunnel syndrome (CTS) include:

   A. Pain in the forearm
   B. Positive Phalen sign
   C. Weakness of thumb flexion
   D. Normal triceps reflex
   E. All of the above

5. _____ Age-related changes which occur in the spine and may be imaged by MRI findings include:

   A. Increase in water content of intervertebral disk
   B. Increase in glycoproteins of intervertebral disk
   C. Increase in height of vertebral bodies
   D. Reduced caliber of spinal canal
   E. All of the above

6. _____ The pathophysiological mechanisms which initiate disk herniation include:

   A. Radial tear of annulus fibrosis
   B. Prolapse of disk
   C. Extrusion of disk
   D. Biochemical changes within disk
   E. All of the above

7. _____ Facet joint degeneration (osteoarthropathy) results from:

   A. Mechanical load and stress resulting from disk space narrowing
   B. Lumbar stenosis
   C. Spine instability
   D. Paget disease
   E. All of the above

8. _____ Approximately this percentage of patients with acute low back pain respond to conservative therapy within 4 weeks:

   A. 50%
   B. 66%
   C. 75%
   D. 90%
   E. 100%

9. _____ If the patient has low back and hip pain and the pain can be exacerbated by external hip rotation, the most likely source of the pain is:

   A. L-4 radiculopathy
   B. Sacro-iliac joint
   C. Hip joint pathology
   D. Lateral femoral cutaneous neuropathy
   E. None of the above

10. _____ In a patient with midthoracic back pain who reports tenderness to palpation over the T-6 vertebral body, the most likely diagnosis is:

   A. Thoracic disk herniation
   B. Metastatic neoplasm
   C. Facet osteoarthropathy
   D. Rheumatoid arthritis
   E. Epidural hematoma

11. _____ A 36-year-old man is evaluated for low back pain of 2 weeks' duration. He is entirely healthy, and the pain occurred after he worked in his garden. This diagnostic study should be done immediately:

   A. EMG/NCV
   B. Plain lumbo-sacral spine radiogram
   C. Myelogram with postmyelogram CT
   D. None of the above
   E. All of the above

12. _____ In patients with neoplastic conus medullaris compression, clinical features usually include:

   A. Symmetrical paraplegia with analgesia at waist level
   B. Normal ankle jerks
   C. Bladder dysfunction
   D. Plantar flexor signs
   E. All of the above

13. _____ In patients with cauda equina compression, clinical features usually include:

   A. Asymmetric leg weakness
   B. Absent ankle and knee reflexes
   C. Bladder dysfunction
   D. All of the above
   E. None of the above

14. _____ The term *spinal shock* refers to:

   A. Depression of spinal reflex activity below the level of injury
   B. Blood loss and hypovolemia following systemic injury
   C. Loss of motor function following spinal injury
   D. Loss of bladder function following spinal injury
   E. All of the above

15. _____ The spinal cord region responsible for reflexogenic penile erection is the:

   A. Parasympathetic center at S-2 to S-4
   B. Sympathetic center at S-2 to S-4
   C. Sympathetic center at T-10 to L-2
   D. Somatic motor fibers at S-2 to S-4
   E. Hypothalamus

16. _____ In a patient with erectile dysfunction, the best test to determine organicity of this disturbance is:

   A. EMG/NCV
   B. Myelogram
   C. Nocturnal penile tumescence (NPT)
   D. Cystometrogram
   E. Endocrine studies

17. _____ Sexual dysfunction occurs in these conditions:

   A. Depressive illness
   B. Diabetes mellitus
   C. Multiple sclerosis
   D. Lumbar sympathectomy
   E. All of the above

Matching

Match the clinical findings with the spinal cord dysfunction.

   A. Immediate paralysis and anesthesia below the lesion with hypotonia and areflexia
   B. Ipsilateral paresis and impairment of vibration and position sense with contralateral pain and temperature impairment
   C. Weakness more marked in arms than in legs, with patchy sensory loss below the level of the lesion
   D. Paralysis with impairment of pin prick below the lesion, with normal vibration and position sense
   E. Pain and paresthesias in the neck, upper arms, and legs, with mild arm weakness and no abnormal corticospinal tract signs

18. _____ Posterior spinal artery syndrome

19. _____ Spinal shock

20. _____ Central cervical cord syndrome

21. _____ Brown-Sequard syndrome

22. _____ Anterior spinal artery syndrome

Multiple Choice

Respond based on the clinical history given.

A 20-year-old man develops difficulty opening jars and manipulating a screwdriver. He has numbness in the forearm and shoulder region. He has no back pain, gait disorder, or bladder symptoms. On examination, he has marked wasting of both hands, with prominent weakness and fasciculations with pin prick impairment over anterior neck and upper forearms, and plantar flexor responses.

23. _____ What location of lesion might cause these findings?

    A. Cervical radiculopathy
    B. Cervical myelopathy
    C. Extradural cervical cord lesion
    D. Intradural extramedullary cervical cord lesion
    E. Intradural intramedullary cervical spinal cord lesion

24. _____ What is the most likely pathological lesion?

    A. Multiple sclerosis
    B. Syringomyelia
    C. Neurofibroma
    D. Meningioma
    E. Metastases

25. _____ What is the most useful diagnostic test?

    A. Lumbar puncture
    B. Myelogram
    C. Postmyelogram CT
    D. Cervical CT
    E. Noncontrast spinal MRI

A 50-year-old man develops back pain and urinary incontinence. Examination shows absent ankle jerks, sensory impairment in the feet and perianal region, weakness of plantar flexion of the feet, and plantar flexor response.

26. _____ What is the location of the lesion causing these findings?

    A. Peripheral neuropathy
    B. Lumbar radiculopathy
    C. Cauda equina lesion
    D. Conus medullaris lesion
    E. All of the above except "A"

27. _____ Which diagnostic test might be useful?

    A. EMG/NCV
    B. Cystometrogram
    C. Lumbar puncture
    D. Myelogram
    E. All of the above

28. _____ If lumbar puncture shows pleocytosis with elevated protein, consider this diagnosis:

    A. Carcinomatous meningitis
    B. Multiple sclerosis
    C. Guillain-Barré syndrome
    D. AIDS-related meningitis
    E. Progressive multifocal leukoencephalopathy

True or False

29. _____ Following MVA with suspected head and neck injury, head CT should not be performed until a screening cervical spine radiogram shows no cervical spine instability.

30. _____ With L4-5 disk herniation, foot dorsiflexors may be weak.

31. _____ With L3-4 disk herniation, the quadriceps muscle is weak and knee jerk is diminished.

32. _____ A ruptured cervical intervertebral disk is most likely to cause C-6 and C-7 symptoms.

33. _____ A ruptured lumbar intervertebral disk is most likely to cause L-5 and S-1 symptoms.

RESPONSES AND EXPLANATIONS

1. **B.** Following a motor vehicle accident, flexion-extension injury with soft tissue musculoskeletal tissue involvement is most common. This causes muscle spasm with loss of cervical lordosis and limitation of lateral rotation. This is called *acute cervical strain syndrome*. The lack of extremity motor, sensory, and reflex neurological abnormalities excludes myelopathy and radiculopathy. Cervical spondylosis is the neurological manifestation of arthritis, and clinical features would include myelopathy and radiculopathy. In SAH, neck flexion impairment is greater than lateral rotation limitation. *(Ref. 1, pp. 27–28; Ref. 2, pp. 610–611; Ref. 4, pp. 24–25)*

2. **A.** With S-1 radiculopathy, there is reduction of ankle reflex due to gastrocnemius muscle weakness. Dorsiflexion of foot is normal, as this involves the L-4 and L-5 roots. Neurogenic bladder is seen with spinal cord or S-2, S-3, and S-4 root involvement. Babinski sign is seen with spinal cord, not spinal root lesions. *(Ref. 1, p. 448; Ref. 2, pp. 596–597)*

3. **E.** A herniated T-8 thoracic disk may compress the thoracic spinal cord, causing all the listed neurological disturbances. It can also cause thoracic radiculopathy resulting in bandlike sensory disturbance in the thoracic or abdominal region. This latter pattern may simulate shingles (herpes zoster without rash). *(Ref. 1, pp. 449–450)*

4. **E.** CTS may simulate C-7 cervical radiculopathy. In cervical radiculopathy, there would be neck pain and reduced triceps reflex. In CTS, pain is usually in the wrist and thumb but may extend to the forearm. In CTS, Tinel sign (tapping over the demyelinated median nerve at the wrist) and Phalen sign (forced wrist flexion causing sensory symptoms in median nerve distribution) are positive. *(Ref. 2, pp. 596–597)*

5. **D.** With advancing age, there is reduced caliber of the spinal canal due to arthritic changes. There is *decreased* water and glycoprotein content of intervertebral disks, with decreased height of vertebral bodies. *(Ref. 1, pp. 455–456; Ref. 2, p. 590)*

6. **A.** Trauma-induced radial tears in the annulus appear to initiate disk herniation. These may be imaged with high-resolution spinal MRI. With normal aging, disk desiccation may occur without disk herniation. *(Ref. 1, pp. 455–456)*

7. **A.** Not all patients with back pain due to arthritic etiology have a herniated disk. There may be arthritic changes which occur in the superior and inferior articular facets that result in back pain. *(Ref. 1, pp. 455–456; Ref. 2, pp. 586–588)*

8. **C.** Seventy to eighty percent of patients who injure their back and report back pain will respond to rest, heat, analgesics, muscle relaxants, and nonsteroidal antiinflammatory medication. Unless the patient appears systemically ill (history of cancer, immunosuppressed status), there is no need to perform any neurodiagnostic studies for at least 4–8 weeks unless there are atypical features (spine tenderness) or evidence of spinal cord dysfunction. *(Ref. 2, pp. 24–31)*

9. **C.** If back pain is exacerbated by stretch signs (straight-leg raising test), consider nerve root compression. If it is exacerbated by tenderness over the sacral-iliac joint, consider local bursitis. If pain is exacerbated by external rotation of the hip, consider hip pathology. Also, consider visceral pathology (kidney, stomach, pancreas, aorta, colon) as the cause of back pain. *(Ref. 2, p. 584)*

10. **B.** Local spine tenderness elicited when palpating directly over the vertebral body is highly suggestive of vertebral body *neoplasm* or infection. Neoplastic conditions or infectious-inflammatory disorders (osteomyelitis) may distend the periosteum, causing local tenderness. This discrete local tenderness should be differentiated from more diffuse muscle spasm seen with a herniated disk. *(Ref. 2, pp. 584–585)*

11. **D.** Due to the paucity of risk factors and normal neurological examination, brief duration of back pain would warrant only symptomatic treatment and no neurodiagnostic studies. *(Ref. 4, pp. 24–31)*

12. **A.** With conus medullaris lesion, the lowest portion of the spinal cord would be involved; therefore there would be leg weakness with upper motor neuron signs (plantar *extensor* signs) with *early* autonomic signs and *loss* of ankle reflexes. *(Ref. 1, p. 413; Ref. 2, pp. 593–594)*

13. **D.** With cauda equina compression, multiple nerve roots are involved. Findings are asymmetrical and autonomic dysfunction occurs *late,* since the spinal cord is not compressed. *(Ref. 1, p. 449; Ref. 2, pp. 593–594)*

14. **A.** Immediately following spinal cord injury, there is electrical-chemical change which enhances inhibitory neurotransmission such that all reflexes are absent. Later, reflexes become hyperreflexive. In adults, spine or brain traumatic injuries do not cause blood loss. With traumatic spinal cord injury, autonomic function occurs immediately, and these patients require catheterization. *(Ref. 1, pp. 440–446)*

15. **A.** Penile erection as well as bladder (micturition) and rectum (defecation) emptying are controlled by parasympathetic (PS) outflow through S-2 to S-4 (pelvic nerves). Acetylcholine is the primary postganglionic PS neurotransmitter. Sympathetic fibers originating at T-10 through L-2 play a central role in seminal emission and ejaculation and are involved in retention of urine and feces. *(Ref. 6, pp. 237–240)*

16. **C.** NPT is the best study to assess erectile dysfunction, whereas a cystometrogram is most useful for assessing abnormalities possibly related to a neurogenic bladder. *(Ref. 6, pp. 237–240)*

17. **E.** Sexual dysfunction occurs in all these conditions. Depression as well as medications used to treat depression should be considered as causal factors. MS causes spinal cord dysfunction and depression, and both conditions lead to sexual dysfunction. Diabetes may cause autonomic neuropathy with sexual dysfunction. *(Ref. 6, pp. 237–240)*

18. **E**

19. **A**

20. **C**

21. **B**

22. **D**

18–22. With posterior spinal artery syndrome, proprioception and vibration sensibility are involved to a greater degree than lateral corticospinal tract dysfunction. With anterior spinal artery syndrome, the opposite is true, such that vibration and position sense are normal. With spinal shock, paralysis and anesthesia with loss of reflexes occur due to enhanced inhibitory neurotransmission. In central cervical cord syndrome, the hands and arms are maximally affected and there is relative leg sparing. With hemisection of the cord (Brown-Sequard syndrome), there is a crossed pattern with loss of pain and temperature (decussate in spinal cord) contralateral to the lesion and impaired ipsilateral motor, vibration, and proprioception findings (both dorsal columns and corticospinal tracts decussate in the brainstem). *(Ref. 2, pp. 165–168)*

23. **E.** Shawl-like sensory impairment involving both shoulders and upper arms indicates impairment of the *central* cord where spinothalamic fibers decussate. Motor dysfunction is due to anterior horn cell involvement. Lack of pain tends to exclude an extradural lesion such as is seen in cervical spondylosis. Lack of autonomic dysfunction, e.g., normal bladder function, is inconsistent with extradural or extramedullary lesion. This pattern is most consistent with *intradural intramedullary lesions* such as syrinx. *(Ref. 2, pp. 602–604)*

24. **B.** Syringomyelia and astrocytoma are the most common lesions. Neurofibroma and meningioma are intradural extramedullary lesions which would compress the cord from outside. Metastases would be extradural lesions and usually cause back pain. MS usually presents with transverse myelitis and symptoms develop acutely. *(Ref. 2, pp. 602–603)*

25. **E.** Noncontrast MRI is most sensitive, as it shows fluid-containing syrinx cavities. There may be neoplasm associated with syrinx, and gadolinium-enhanced spinal MRI should be done if syrinx is present. *(Ref. 1, pp. 750–753)*

26. **E.** It is important to recognize that autonomic dysfunction and *perineal* region sensory dysfunction *rarely* both occur with peripheral neuropathy. In diabetic and amyloid neuropathy, autonomic neuropathy may cause bladder or bowel dysfunction. The perineal nerves are *short* nerves, and *long* nerves are affected by neuropathy. *(Ref. 1, p. 161)*

27. **D.** Since a mass lesion involving the lower spinal cord region is suspected, neuro-imaging of this region with myelogram, MRI, or CT should be performed. *(Ref. 2, pp. 62–63)*

28. **A.** Also consider carcinomatous or lymphomatous meningitis. If CSF shows pleocytosis, perform cytology to determine if the cells are neoplastic. *(Ref. 1, p. 354)*

29. **T.** Prior to performing brain CT in which the neck must be extended, the middle and lower cervical spine must be assessed for instability. Remember that patients with suspected head injury may also have spine injury. *(Ref. 2, pp. 606–610)*

30. **T.** At this level, the L-5 root is compressed. Both L-4 and L-5 roots supply foot dorsiflexors. Due to dual innervation of foot dorsiflexors, clinical examination may show no weakness if only one root is compressed; however, EMG may show some denervation changes which are present but not severe enough to cause clinical weakness. *(Ref. 1, p. 448; Ref. 2, pp. 596–597)*

31. **T.** At this level, the L-4 root is compressed to cause these changes. *(Ref. 1, p. 448; Ref. 2, pp. 596–597)*

32. **T.** In the cervical region, the C-6 root exists between the C-5 and C-6 vertebral bodies and the C-7 root exits between the C-6 and C-7 vertebral bodies. At these levels, there is maximal spinal mobility. *(Ref. 1, p. 448; Ref. 2, pp. 596–597)*

33. **T.** In the lumbar region, L-5 roots exit between L-4 and L-5 vertebral bodies and S-1 roots exit between L-5 and S-1 vertebral bodies. These are regions of maximal spinal mobility. Disk herniation is most likely to occur at these regions. *(Ref. 1, p. 448; Ref. 2, pp. 596–597)*

6

CEREBROVASCULAR DISEASE

True or False

1. _____ In patients with transient ischemic attack (TIA), neurological deficit lasts more than 24 hr but less than 72 hr.

2. _____ In patients with stroke syndrome, neurological deficit comes on gradually and takes 1–3 days to reach maximal severity.

3. _____ Hypertension and cardiac disease are major risk factors for stroke.

4. _____ Lacunar infarcts are characteristic of hypertensive cerebrovascular disease; two common clinical patterns of lacunes are pure sensory stroke and Wallenberg syndrome.

5. _____ Anterior cerebral artery (ACA) territory infarctions cause contralateral leg weakness and sensory impairment.

6. _____ In patients with nonvalvular atrial fibrillation, aspirin is more effective than anticoagulation for stroke prevention.

7. _____ In asymptomatic patients with 60% stenosis of the intracranial portion of the carotid artery, carotid endarterectomy (CEA) is warranted.

Multiple Choice

Choose the appropriate response.

8. _____ If a chronic hypertensive man died suddenly of myocardial infarction but never had clinical stroke, autopsy may commonly show this finding:

    A. Mycotic aneurysm
    B. Ectatic aneurysm
    C. Berry aneurysm
    D. Charcot-Bouchard aneurysm
    E. C and D

9. _____ Which of the following is common in stroke patients, and its occurrence interferes with rehabilitative efforts:

    A. Anosagnosia of Babinski
    B. Visual field defect
    C. Urinary incontinence
    D. Thalamic pain syndrome
    E. Atrial fibrillation

10. _____ The following location(s) are characteristic of hypertensive intracerebral hemorrhages (ICH):

    A. Basal ganglia (globus pallidus)
    B. Pons (dorsal)
    C. Internal capsule
    D. Thalamus
    E. All of the above

11. _____ If a patient has a 15-min episode of aphasia and right hemiparesis and CT is normal and carotid angiogram shows 70% stenosis of the left extracranial internal carotid artery, appropriate treatment would be:

    A. Carotid endarterectomy (CEA)
    B. Intravenous heparin
    C. Coumadin
    D. High-dose aspirin
    E. Ticlopidine

12. _____ If the patient has carotid bruit, which statements are correct?

    A. Patient must have carotid stenosis
    B. Risk of stroke is 6% per year
    C. Carotid endarterectomy is indicated
    D. Risk of myocardial infarction justifies cardiac evaluation
    E. Carotid Doppler duplex ultrasound should be performed as next procedure to determine the presence and degree of arterial stenosis

13. _____ The following is an uncommon mechanism of nonlacunar ischemic stroke:

    A. Cardiogenic cerebral embolism
    B. Artery-to-artery embolism
    C. Hypoperfusion
    D. Thrombosis *in situ*
    E. None of the above

14. _____ The most common major potential side effect of ticlopidine is:

A. Skin rash
B. Diarrhea
C. Irreversible neutropenia
D. Reversible neutropenia
E. Liver failure

15. _____ Conditions which may lead to worsening neurological deficit in acute stroke patients include:

A. Hypoxia
B. Hyperthermia
C. Hyperglycemia
D. Atrial fibrillation (AF)
E. All of the above

16. _____ Clinical features of left posterior cerebral artery (PCA) occlusion include:

A. Right homonymous hemianopsia and hemianesthesia
B. Right hemiballismus
C. Vertigo and ataxia
D. Right hemiparesis
E. Alexia with agraphia

17. _____ The following deficiencies or disease states are associated with venous sinus thrombosis (VST):

A. Protein S
B. Protein C
C. Antithrombin III
D. Sickle cell disease
E. All of the above

18. _____ Clinical lacunar stroke syndromes include:

A. Pure motor hemiparesis
B. Pure sensory hemianesthesia
C. Dysarthria–clumsy hand syndrome
D. Crural ataxia–hemiparesis
E. All of the above

19. _____ A potential common cause of nonhypertensive brain hemorrhage is:

A. Meningioma
B. Brain abscess
C. Subdural hematoma
D. Cocaine
E. Marijuana

20. _____ This is one of the effects of aspirin:

A. Decreases bleeding time
B. Increases prothrombin time

C. Increases partial thromboplastin time
D. Acetylates platelet cyclooxygenase to decrease thromboxane synthesis
E. Impairs fibrinogen function

21. _____ This medication has been shown effective in secondary stroke prevention in noncardiogenic stroke:

A. Aspirin
B. Ticlopidine
C. Dipyridamole
D. Coumadin
E. All of the above

22. _____ Effective therapy for stroke-induced edema is:

A. Osmotic agents
B. Diuretics
C. Corticosteroids
D. Acetazolamide
E. None of the above

23. _____ The clinical syndrome associated with superior cerebellar artery (SCA) infarction is:

A. Ipsilateral ataxia
B. Horner syndrome
C. Contralateral anesthesia
D. Ipsilateral chorea
E. All of the above

24. _____ The following visual findings occur in patients with central retinal artery occlusion (CRAO):

A. Unilateral amaurosis
B. Retinal edema
C. Cherry red spot
D. Optic atrophy
E. All of the above

25. _____ Following subarachnoid hemorrhage (SAH), this is a common metabolic derangement:

A. Metabolic acidosis
B. Respiratory acidosis
C. Hyponatremia
D. Hypokalemia
E. Hypercalcemia

26. _____ Neurological deterioration following aneurysmal SAH may be due to:

A. Cerebral ischemia
B. Hydrocephalus
C. Rebleeding
D. Vasospasm
E. All of the above

27. _____ This treatment is effective in acute carotid artery occlusion:

  A. Emergency carotid endarterectomy
  B. Superficial temporal-middle cerebral artery bypass
  C. Calcium channel blockers
  D. Angioplasty
  E. None of the above

28. _____ In a 50-year-old man with an asymptomatic carotid bruit due to high-grade carotid stenosis, this is the most common cause of death:

  A. Myocardial infarction
  B. Cerebral infarction
  C. Cerebral hemorrhage
  D. Pulmonary embolism
  E. Subarachnoid hemorrhage

29. _____ The following is approved indication for extracranial-intracranial bypass surgery:

  A. Intracranial carotid stenosis
  B. Vasospasm due to giant intracranial aneurysm
  C. Moyamoya disease
  D. Carotid dissection
  E. None of the above

30. _____ Factors altering blood viscosity include:

  A. Hematocrit
  B. Fibrinogen
  C. Erythrocyte aggregabililty and deformabililty
  D. Platelet aggregation
  E. All of the above

31. _____ Cerebral venous thrombosis (CVT) most commonly occurs during:

  A. Pregnancy
  B. Puerperium
  C. Menopause
  D. Menarche
  E. In patients utilizing low-dose estrogen oral contraceptive medication

32. _____ Diagnosis of cerebral venous thrombosis is definitively established by the following studies:

  A. Conventional catheter angiography
  B. MRI
  C. Postcontrast CT
  D. SPECT
  E. Transcranial Doppler

33. _____ Potential causes of stroke in migraine patients include:

  A. Ergot intoxication
  B. Reversible vasoconstrictive angiopathy
  C. Oral contraceptive medication
  D. Antiphospholipid antibody syndrome (APLAS)
  E. All of the above

34. _____ Primary antiphospholipid antibody syndrome includes these clinical features:

  A. Spontaneous abortion
  B. Deep venous thrombosis
  C. Stroke syndromes
  D. Cardiac lesions
  E. All of the above

35. _____ Neurological complications resulting from cardiac surgery may be due to this mechanism:

  A. Air and particulate microembolism
  B. Cardiogenic cerebral embolism
  C. Hypotension
  D. All of the above
  E. None of the above

36. _____ The following statement is true of serum lipid levels and stroke:

  A. Serum cholesterol level below 160 mg/dL is associated with increased incidence of intracerebral and subarachnoid hemorrhage
  B. Atherosclerosis of carotid artery is usually related to serum cholesterol levels
  C. There is a direct correlation between myocardial and brain infarctions of all types with serum cholesterol level
  D. All of the above
  E. None of the above

From the clinical history, choose the most appropriate response.

A 50-year-old normotensive man has an episode of sudden loss of vision in the right eye. This persists for 15 min and then rapidly resolves. He has normal neurological and ophthalmological examination.

37. _____ The mechanism of this episode is most likely:

  A. Demyelination of optic nerve
  B. Artery-to-artery embolism involving carotid and ophthalmic arteries
  C. Thrombosis *in situ* in carotid artery
  D. Optic nerve compression
  E. None of the above

38. _____ The most cost-effective diagnostic test would be:

   A. CT with contrast
   B. MR with gadolinium
   C. Doppler duplex ultrasound
   D. Catheter cerebral angiogram
   E. None of the above

39. _____ Likely differential diagnostic considerations include:

   A. Migraine equivalent
   B. Antiphospholipid antibody syndrome (APLAS)
   C. Optic neuritis
   D. Cardiogenic cerebral embolism
   E. None of the above

40. _____ A possible accompanying neurological sign in this patient might be:

   A. Transcortical motor aphasia
   B. Anosagnosia of Babinski
   C. Anton syndrome
   D. Thalamic pain syndrome
   E. Cerebellar ataxia

41. _____ Effective therapy might include:

   A. Timoptic
   B. Coumadin
   C. Ticlid
   D. Aspirin
   E. Cannot determine based on given information

A 50-year-old man with atrial fibrillation suddenly becomes "confused." He is alert and attentive. His speech is fluent but he has difficulty following commands.

42. _____ The following other neurological examination abnormalities might be seen:

   A. Hemiparesis
   B. Homonymous hemianopsia
   C. Anomia
   D. Agraphia
   E. No focal findings, since patient has encephalopathy

43. _____ Initial diagnostic study should include:

   A. Drug screen
   B. Biochemical profile
   C. EKG and EEG
   D. CT
   E. MRI

44. _____ Initial treatment should be:

   A. Aspirin
   B. Ticlopidine
   C. Persantine
   D. Heparin
   E. Coumadin

A 54-year-old hypertensive man develops headache, vomits, and becomes confused. Examination shows lethargy, right hemiparesis, and right hemianesthesia with head and eyes deviated to the left. Blood pressure is 210/120 mmHg.

45. _____ The most likely diagnosis is:

   A. Subarachnoid hemorrhage
   B. Middle cerebral artery occlusion
   C. Carotid occlusion
   D. Hypertensive encephalopathy
   E. Putaminal hemorrhage

46. _____ The most cost-effective diagnostic test is:

   A. LP
   B. MRI
   C. Noncontrast CT
   D. Cerebral angiogram
   E. Carotid Doppler

47. _____ Treatment should include:

   A. Nimodipine
   B. Heparin
   C. Corticosteroids
   D. Carotid endarterectomy
   E. None of the above

A 52-year-old hypertensive, diabetic man awakens unable to speak coherently and has right arm and face weakness but the leg is not affected. Examination shows dysarthria, Broca aphasia, right hemiparesis (face and arm), and hemianesthesia. Blood pressure is 220/110 mmHg.

48. _____ The most likely diagnosis is:

   A. Left putaminal hemorrhage
   B. Left middle cerebral artery (MCA) occlusion
   C. Left carotid occlusion
   D. Left anterior cerebral artery occlusion
   E. Left posterior cerebral artery occlusion

49. _____ The most cost-effective diagnostic study is:

   A. Noncontrast CT
   B. Postcontrast CT
   C. MRI
   D. LP
   E. Carotid Doppler ultrasound

50. _____ Initial treatment should include:

   A. Rapid lowering of blood pressure to 120/80 mmHg
   B. Hyperventilation
   C. Heparin
   D. Ticlid
   E. None of the above

A 50-year-old hypertensive man develops headache and vomits. He becomes confused and has a generalized seizure. Examination shows lethargy, bilateral plantar extensor responses, and hypertensive retinopathy. Blood pressure is 260/140 mmHg.

51. _____ The most likely diagnosis is:

   A. Hypertensive encephalopathy
   B. Subarachnoid hemorrhage
   C. Intracerebral hemorrhage
   D. Subdural hematoma
   E. Brain neoplasm with transtentorial herniation

52. _____ The most useful diagnostic study is:

   A. Noncontrast CT
   B. Postcontrast CT
   C. LP
   D. Angiogram
   E. MRI

53. _____ The most appropriate treatment is:

   A. Sublingual nimodipine
   B. Sublingual nitroglycerin
   C. Intravenous nitroprusside
   D. Intravenous hydralazine
   E. Intravenous dexamethasone

54. _____ Potential complications of this neurological disorder include:

   A. Myocardial ischemia
   B. Congestive heart failure
   C. Renal failure
   D. All of the above
   E. None of the above

A 60-year-old hypertensive, Afro-American woman awakens unable to use her left arm and drags her left leg. Examination shows pure motor hemiparesis. Blood pressure is 160/100 mmHg.

55. _____ The most likely diagnosis is:

   A. Right capsular infarct
   B. Right thalamic infarct
   C. Lateral medullary infarct
   D. Anterior cerebral artery territory infarct
   E. None of the above

56. _____ The most useful diagnostic test is:

   A. CT
   B. SPECT
   C. LP
   D. Angiogram
   E. MRI

57. _____ Treatment to prevent stroke recurrence should include:

   A. Intravenous Heparin
   B. Ticlid
   C. Aspirin
   D. Carotid endarterectomy
   E. Coumadin

A 58-year-old hypertensive man awakens feeling dizzy, vomits, and has occipital headache. Exam shows broad-based ataxic gait with impaired heel-to-shin but normal finger-to-nose movements. There is right lateral rectus paresis and horizontal nystagmus. Blood pressure is 180/110 mmHg.

58. _____ The most likely diagnosis is:

   A. Vestibular neuronitis
   B. Cerebellar hemorrhage
   C. Pontine hemorrhage
   D. Thalamic hemorrhage
   E. None of the above

59. _____ Initial diagnostic study should be:

   A. MRI
   B. LP
   C. Noncontrast CT
   D. Postcontrast CT
   E. Angiogram

60. _____ Treatment should include:

   A. Nitroprusside to lower blood pressure
   B. Dexamethasone to reduce cerebral edema
   C. Heparin to reduce clot propagation
   D. Emergency surgery to remove hematoma
   E. None of the above

61. _____ The most likely location of the lesion causing the neurological deficit is the:

   A. Vermis of cerebellum
   B. Cerebellar hemisphere
   C. Pons
   D. Midbrain
   E. Thalamus

Within 30 min, the patient became confused, blood pressure increased to 240/140 mmHg, pulse became 40 beats/min, and respiration slowed to 6/min.

62. _____ Diagnostic considerations include:

    A. Tonsillar herniation
    B. Subfalcine herniation
    C. Transtentorial herniation
    D. Uncal herniation
    E. None of the above

63. _____ The neural substrate which is affected to cause these neurological changes might include:

    A. Secondary brainstem compression
    B. Hypertensive encephalopathy
    C. Vasospasm
    D. All of the above
    E. None of the above

64. _____ Treatment would include:

    A. Hyperventilation
    B. Mannitol
    C. Glycerol
    D. Surgical decompression
    E. All of the above

A 24-year-old man develops sudden onset of left-sided headache and vomits. He then has a generalized seizure. Exam shows confusion, with difficulty comprehending speech and right homonymous hemianopsia.

65. _____ The location of the lesion causing the neurological disturbance is likely to be the:

    A. Left temporal lobe
    B. Left parietal lobe
    C. Left frontal lobe
    D. Right temporal lobe
    E. None of the above

66. _____ The most likely pathological condition causing this neurological presentation is:

    A. Glioma
    B. Intracerebral hematoma
    C. Cerebral infarction
    D. Meningioma
    E. Herpes simplex encephalitis

67. _____ Initial diagnostic study should be:

    A. CT
    B. LP
    C. MRI
    D. Angiogram
    E. EEG

68. _____ Definitive diagnostic study would be:

    A. CT
    B. MRI
    C. LP
    D. Angiogram
    E. EEG

69. _____ The most likely etiology of the visualized hemorrhage would be:

    A. Hypertension
    B. Amyloid
    C. Arteriovenous malformation
    D. Neoplasm
    E. Aneurysm

A 50-year-old mildly hypertensive, ectomorphic man who has no prior cardiovascular or cerebrovascular symptoms is found to have a left carotid bruit. Neurological examination is entirely normal.

70. _____ Initial diagnostic study should be:

    A. Carotid duplex Doppler ultrasound
    B. CT
    C. MRI
    D. Conventional carotid angiogram
    E. MR angiogram

71. _____ The presence of carotid bruit indicates:

    A. Carotid stenosis
    B. Turbulent arterial flow
    C. Carotid occlusion
    D. Aortic valve disease
    E. None of the above

72. _____ If vascular imaging studies shows 70% carotid stenosis, this therapeutic intervention would be warranted:

    A. Carotid endarterectomy
    B. Low-dose aspirin
    C. High-dose aspirin
    D. Ticlopidine
    E. Coumadin

73. _____ If MRI shows three high-intensity, small round lesions in the basal ganglia, these indicate the following pathological disturbances:

A. Enlarged perivascular spaces
B. Multiple sclerosis
C. Lacunar hemorrhages
D. Hemodynamic ischemic lesions
E. Arterial border-zone infarcts

74. _____ To be effective for stroke prevention, risk of carotid endarterectomy should be less than this percentage:

A. 3%
B. 5%
C. 7%
D. 9%
E. 15%

RESPONSES AND EXPLANATIONS

1. **F.** Definition of TIA requires that "ministroke" lasts *less* than 24 hr; however, the *majority* of TIAs last *less* than 30 minutes. In reversible ischemic neurological deficit (RIND), deficit lasts longer than 24 hr but usually less than 1 week. Remember that stroke classification based on temporal pattern, e.g., TIA, RIND, is meaningless from therapeutic perspective. It is important to know the underlying vascular (arterial) lesion to determine appropriate treatment strategy. *(Ref. 4, pp.118–121)*

2. **F.** The definition of stroke is *sudden* onset of *focal* neurological deficit. This reaches *maximal* severity rapidly; however, in some patients, their condition may worsen over a several-hour interval (*progressive* or *deteriorating* stroke). Approximately 25% of patients die of stroke within the initial 30 days. *(Ref. 4, pp. 124–131)*

3. **T.** Hypertension is a major risk factor for both hemorrhagic and ischemic stroke. Cardiac disease is a major risk factor for embolic disease. *(Ref. 1, p. 253)*

4. **F.** Lacunar infarcts are due to lipohyalinosis and fibrinoid degeneration of arterioles, most characteristically occurring in hypertensive patients. This arteriolar occlusion is angiographically *invisible*. Pure sensory stroke is due to lacunar disease; however, Wallenberg syndrome is due to *large* vessel (arterial) disease due to either vertebral or posterior inferior cerebellar arterial occlusion. *(Ref. 2, pp. 282–284)*

5. **T.** ACA occlusion causes motor and sensory deficit in the *contralateral* leg with *sparing* of face and arm. Face and arm motor and sensory representations are located on the lateral surface of the hemisphere in the *middle* cerebral artery territory. Leg motor and sensory representations are located in the medial parasagittal region in distribution of ACA. *(Ref. 2, p. 273)*

6. **F.** There is consensus that anticoagulation is more effective than aspirin in stroke prevention in atrial fibrillation. With low-dose oral anticoagulation, the risk of hemorrhage is 1–2%. *(New England Journal of Medicine 323, pp. 1505–1510, 1990; Journal of the American College of Cardiologists 18, pp. 349–356, 1991; Ref. 2, pp. 268–270)*

7. **F.** CEA is warranted with 60% or greater stenosis of the *extracranial* portion of the carotid artery. CEA is superior to antiplatelet or anticoagulant medication. In asymptomatic patients, CEA had lower complication rate in men than in women; therefore the benefit of CEA is greater in men than in women. *(Journal of the American Medical Association 273, p. 1421, 1995)*

8. **D.** Charcot-Bouchard aneurysms develop within arterioles of chronic hypertensive patients; these are sources of hypertensive intracerebral hematomas. Berry aneurysms occur at branch points of arteries and are sources of subarachnoid hemorrhage. Mycotic aneurysms are due to infectious etiology and may develop in patients with bacterial endocarditis. Ectatic aneurysms are dilations of arteries due to atherosclerotic disease and cause thickening of arterial walls, resulting in cerebral infarction, *not* hemorrhage. *(Ref. 2, p. 285)*

9. **A.** Anosagnosia of Babinski refers to denial of left-sided motor deficit; this occurs with right parietal lesions. Some patients neglect or are inattentive to their hemiparetic left side. This means that these patients are unlikely to participate actively in their rehabilitation efforts. Special neurorehabilitation techniques must be utilized in these patients to overcome neglect and inattention. *(Ref. 2, p. 270)*

10. **D.** These ICH are usually located in
    a. Basal ganglia (*putamen*)
    b. Pons (involving ventral *and* tegmental [dorsal] regions)
    c. Cerebellum
    d. Thalamus
    ICH may extend *across* the internal capsule. *(Ref. 1, pp. 256–257; Ref. 2, pp. 285–290)*

11. **A.** In patients who experience TIA and have 70% stenosis of the *extracranial* carotid artery, CEA would be warranted. This assumes the patient has no complicating medical conditions. While awaiting surgery, intravenous anticoagulation should be utilized to avoid stroke occurrence. *(New England Journal of Medicine 325, p. 441, 1991)*

12. **E.** Carotid bruit indicates that flow is *turbulent* and *not laminar*. It may occur *without* carotid stenosis. To determine if bruit is due to carotid stenosis, perform noninvasive carotid duplex Doppler ultrasound. *(New England Journal of Medicine 315, p. 860, 1986; Ref. 4, pp. 116–117)*

13. **D.** In patients with coronary artery disease, thrombosis *in situ* is a common mechanism for myocardial infarction; however, for ischemic stroke, *embolism* is more common than thrombosis *in situ*. Hypoperfusion may cause ischemia in arterial borderzones (distal poorly perfused regions between adjacent arterial territories, e.g., ACA and MCA, MCA and PCA). *(Ref. 1, pp. 227–242)*

14. **B.** Diarrhea is the most common minor side effect, which can be controlled by taking medication with meals. The most serious potential side effect is reversible neutropenia which occurs within the initial 3 months of therapy. During this time period, perform a white blood cell count every 2 weeks. *(Lancet 1, p. 86, 1989; New England Journal of Medicine 320, p. 501, 1989)*

15. **E.** AF may cause stroke recurrence. The occurrence of the other factors should be avoided in stroke patients, as they worsen neurological deficit. If infection complicates stroke, e.g., pneumonia, urinary tract infection, treat aggressively, as fever and infection precipitate neurological worsening. *(Ref. 2, pp. 267–268; Ref. 4, pp. 124–125)*

16. **A.** In most patients, right homonymous hemianopsia is the sole finding; however, PCA may supply the thalamus and this may also result in hemianesthesia. Alexia *without* agraphia may result from left PCA territory infarction. *(Ref. 2, p. 273)*

17. **E.** All listed *anticoagulant* factors may cause hypercoagulable state if they are deficient and result in VST. Also, sickle cell disease may result in hypercoagulable state resulting in arterial or venous stroke. *(Ref. 1, pp. 264–271; Ref. 4, pp. 132–133)*

18. **E.** All are characteristic hypertensive lacunar syndromes. Pure motor hemiparesis is due to internal capsule or pontine lacune. Pure sensory stroke is due to thalamic lacune. Dysarthria–clumsy hand syndrome is due to brainstem lacune. The location of the lesion causing ataxia–hemiparesis is not clearly established. *(Ref. 2, pp. 28–35)*

19. **C.** Trauma may cause bleeding of bridging veins; this may lead to SDH. Cocaine has a sympathomimetic effect and may cause *hypertensive* brain hemorrhage. The other conditions are *not* associated with brain hemorrhage. *(Ref. 2, pp. 284–290; Ref. 4, pp. 134–135)*

20. **D.** The major effect of aspirin is to interfere with thromboxane A_2 formation. It *increases* bleeding time. In stroke prevention, aspirin probably also has an effect on endothelial wall function and structure. *(Ref. 2, p. 266)*

21. **B.** In patients who suffer initial completed stroke, ticlopidine has been demonstrated to be effective in preventing stroke recurrence. If the patient has a cardiogenic source of stroke, anticoagulation is effective in preventing stroke recurrence. *(Ref. 2, pp. 266–267)*

22. **E.** For cytotoxic and vasogenic edema which may occur in ischemic or hemorrhagic stroke, no agent has been demonstrated to be effective. *(Ref. 2, pp. 266–267; Ref. 4, pp. 124–125)*

23. **A.** With SCA ischemia, ipsilateral ataxia is the characteristic finding, due to midbrain ischemia (involvement of superior cerebellar peduncle). *(Ref. 2, pp. 276–277)*

24. **E.** The ophthalmic artery is the initial branch of the internal carotid artery. This branches into the central retinal artery. Transient ischemia of the ophthalmic artery may cause unilateral *amaurosis fugax*. With CRAO, retinal ischemia may cause all listed findings. If the arterial occlusion does not resolve, retinal infarct occurs and permanent blindness may result. *(Ref. 1, p. 246; Ref. 2, pp. 270–272)*

25. **C.** Hyponatremia may result from vasopressin or arterial natriuretic factor excess, which frequently develops in patients with SAH. *(Ref. 2, pp. 679–681)*

26. **E.** Following initial bleeding from a berry aneurysm, rebleeding may occur. Blood clots which develop in the subarachnoid space may lead to vasospasm, ischemia, and hydrocephalus. *(Ref. 1, pp. 275–284; Ref. 2, pp. 290–296)*

27. **E.** Once carotid *occlusion* occurs, no type of revascularization procedure is effective. Calcium-channel blockers may reduce blood pressure and *worsen* neurological deficit, due to cerebral hypoperfusion. *(Ref. 2, pp. 270–272)*

28. **A.** In patients with multifocal atherosclerotic disease, myocardial infarction and sudden unexplained vascular death are more common than stroke. This means that patients with carotid bruits should have careful cardiac (coronary artery) evaluation even if they have *no* cardiac symptoms. *(Ref. 2, pp. 251–257)*

29. **E.** Although the theory of the superficial temporal artery-to-middle cerebral artery bypass procedure makes sense from a hemodynamic perspective, clinical studies have shown no benefit. Similar vascular bypass procedures have been attempted within the vertebral-basilar arterial system, but once again there are no studies demonstrating clinical efficacy. *(New England Journal of Medicine 317, p. 1505, 1987)*

30. **E.** By hemodilution (lower hematocrit to 35%), ischemic stroke may be prevented; however, by lowering hematocrit to less than 35%, oxygen-carrying capacity of the blood may be reduced, exacerbating ischemia. Elevated fibrinogen may increase blood viscosity; this may be reduced by ancrod, which is a defibrinating agent. Platelet aggregation is reduced by aspirin or ticlopidine. Trental is utilized to alter RBC deformability and reduce blood viscosity. *(Journal of Neurology, Neurosurgery, and Psychiatry 70, p. 6, 1993)*

31. **B.** At the time of delivery and for several weeks following delivery, CVT may occur. Use of *high-dose (not* low-dose) estrogen may be associated with increased stroke risk. *(Neurologic Clinics of North America 10, p. 87, 1992; Ref. 2, pp. 299–300)*

32. **A.** To image venous sinus thrombosis, an angiogram is warranted. Postcontrast CT may occasionally show venous abnormalities but it is less sensitive than an angiogram. MRI or CT may show venous infarct or hemorrhage but not the underlying vascular abnormalities. Transcranial Doppler shows the *intracranial* arterial system only. *(Ref. 1, pp. 285–289)*

33. **E.** Stroke is *unusual* in migraine patients. The neurological aura is due to a spreading cortical depression (not vasoconstriction) and usually resolves when the headache begins. The use of ergot medication is *not* contraindicated in migraine with aura; however if overdose of ergots is given, vasoconstrictive angiopathy may occur. Risk factors for stroke in migraine patients include hypertension, cigarette smoking, and family history of stroke. APLAS may predispose to stroke. *(Annals of Neurology 26, p. 386, 1989)*

34. **E.** These include lupus anticoagulant and anticardiolipin antibodies. They may cause recurrent thrombotic episodes involving both arterial and venous circulation. Treatment includes suppression of immune-mediated thrombotic response, anticoagulants, or antiplatelet agents. *(Stroke 18, p. 257, 1987)*

35. **D.** Neurological effects of cardiac surgery include *stroke* and *hypoxic ischemic encephalopathy. Microembolization* may result from blood pressure fluctuations and coagulation factor abnormalities. Following surgery, patients may develop memory and subtle neuropsychological disturbances due to these vascular complications. *(Ref. 2, pp. 679–699)*

36. **B.** With coronary artery disease, there is a direct relationship between lipid abnormalities and myocardial infarction. With stroke, the issue is less clear. First, there appears to be a relationship between elevated cholesterol and carotid atherosclerosis such that lovastatin treatment reduces carotid stenosis. Second, there is no demonstrated relationship between small vessel disease and cholesterol level. Third, there appears to be an *unexpected* relationship between cholesterol level and intracerebral hemorrhage, such that high rates of ICH occur in patients with low cholesterol levels. *(Neurologic Clinics of North America 1, p. 317, 1983; Annals of Neurology 26, p. 3, 1989)*

37. **B.** This is TIA referred to as "amaurosis fugax" due to carotid atherosclerotic disease. There is artery-to-artery embolism from the carotid to the ophthalmic to the central retinal artery. This causes sudden transient blindness. Optic nerve demyelination may cause sudden visual loss but would not resolve so quickly, and funduscopic examination would show evidence of disk inflammation (papillitis); compression of the optic nerve would cause *gradual* visual loss with funduscopic evidence of optic pallor and reduced pupillary light response. *(Ref. 1, pp. 58–59)*

38. **D.** With carotid territory TIA, conventional carotid angiogram would be necessary to show the extra- and intracranial portions of the carotid artery. Doppler duplex ultrasound shows only the *extracranial* carotid artery. Since the attack was not referable to cerebral hemispheres, CT or MRI would not be likely to show brain abnormality. *(Ref. 2, pp. 260–263; Ref. 4, pp. 120–121)*

39. **A.** Retinal migraine or migraine equivalent can cause visual loss; however, it is usually followed by headache and visual disturbances which extend across the visual field over an interval of 10–30 min rather than coming on suddenly as in TIA. APLAS may cause migraine-like episodes. *(Ref. 4, pp. 58–59)*

40. **B.** If the right eye is involved, this is due to *right* carotid disease. This causes ischemia of the right hemisphere with *left* hemiparesis and possibly denial or neglect (hemi-inattention) syndrome (anosognosia of Babinski). *(Ref. 2, pp. 270–273)*

41. **E.** To know how to treat this TIA patient to prevent major permanent stroke, it is necessary to know the nature of the underlying vascular lesion. If the extracranial carotid is stenotic, consider CEA. If there is severe rate-limiting stenosis (which is not surgically accessible), consider that there is a "red clot" thrombus formation and utilize Coumadin. If there is ulcerated plaque but no severe rate-limiting stenosis, consider antiplatelet agents (aspirin, Ticlid). *(Ref. 2, pp. 120–121)*

42. **B.** Sudden onset indicates vascular etiology. Because the patient appears confused and cannot comprehend normally, this indicates Wernicke aphasia. This involves the posterior temporal lobe of dominant hemisphere. The visual field fibers pass through this region and ischemia may cause right homonymous hemianopsia. Therefore, patients with Wernicke aphasia have accompanying right homonymous hemianopsia but *no* hemiparesis or hemianesthesia. *(Ref. 1, pp. 8–11; Ref. 2, pp. 268–270)*

43. **D.** CT should be performed to be certain that hemorrhage has not occurred and to determine the presence and size of cerebral ischemic-infarction lesions. *(Neurology 38, p. 791, 1988)*

44. **D.** In cardiogenic cerebral embolism, anticoagulation utilizing heparin should be initiated. There is risk of hemorrhagic transformation within the initial 48 hr following cardiogenic cerebral embolism; however, this must be balanced against the risk of stroke recurrence if heparin is *not* utilized. *(Neurology 38, p. 314, 1988)*

45. **E.** Sudden onset of neurological deficit in a hypertensive patient indicates vascular etiology. Occurrence of headache, vomiting, and confusion are consistent with hemorrhage. The finding of right hemiparesis with horizontal deviation of the eyes to *the opposite* side is consistent with putaminal hemorrhage. With SAH, headache and nuchal rigidity are prominent features. Blood pressure is not high enough to be consistent with hypertensive encephalopathy. *(Ref. 4, pp. 8–15)*

46. **C.** Noncontrast CT would be the initial procedure, as the clinical suspicion is higher for intracerebral hemorrhage than for cerebral ischemia. *(Ref. 1, pp. 243–245)*

47. **E.** With hypertensive hemorrhage, hematoma develops rapidly and blood pressure lowering does not usually help to limit maximal hematoma size. *(Ref. 4, pp. 138–141)*

48. **B.** The distribution of weakness (face and arm with *sparing* of leg) and Broca aphasia suggests ischemia in MCA distribution. With carotid occlusion, the territory of MCA and ACA would be affected such that the face, arm, and leg would be equally affected. Putaminal (subcortical) hemorrhage would not likely cause aphasia. *(Ref. 2, pp. 270–272)*

49. **C.** If an ischemic lesion is suspected, MRI is most sensitive to detect early ischemia changes. *(Ref. 1, pp. 243–245)*

50. **E.** Blood pressure should not be lowered, because this reduction may reduce brain perfusion pressure and this might worsen the neurological deficit. Since there are no signs of intracranial hypertension or cerebral edema, hyperventilation would not be warranted. Ticlopidine is not effective for 72–96 hr; however, aspirin would have immediate effect on platelet aggregation. As neurological deficit is stable and not progressing and there is no evidence of cardiogenic cerebral embolism, heparin would not be warranted. *(Ref. 2, pp. 276–280)*

51. **A.** Acute hypertensive vascular crisis (*hypertensive encephalopathy*) is characterized by rapid blood pressure elevation with *generalized* (nonfocal) neurological signs and funduscopic evidence of hypertensive retinopathy. *(Ref. 4, pp. 154–155)*

52. **A.** This is clinical diagnosis, and *no* diagnostic study is necessary to establish this diagnosis; however, noncontrast CT could be performed to exclude other neurological conditions which might clinically simulate hypertensive encephalopathy. In HE, CT is usually normal but may show white matter ischemic lesions in parietal-occipital regions. *(Ref. 4, pp. 154–155)*

53. **C.** Treatment of HE includes use of antihypertensive agents which allow rapid but monitored controlled blood pressure reduction. Although there may be cerebral edema, corticosteroids are not indicated for HE. *(Neurologic Clinics of North America 1, p. 3, 1985)*

54. **D.** Marked prolonged elevated of blood pressure may cause cardiac and renal ischemia. *(Neurologic Clinics of North America 1, p. 3, 1985)*

55. **A.** Hypertension is a major risk factor for arteriolar disease to cause lacunar infarct. Sudden onset of pure motor hemiparesis involving the arm and leg equally (or the face, arm, and leg) is characteristic of right capsular infarct. *(Ref. 2, pp. 282–285)*

56. **E.** MRI shows small ischemic lesions more sensitively than CT. SPECT may show cortical areas of decreased perfusion, but these hypoperfused areas due to capsular lesions are unlikely to be visualized with SPECT because of their small size. *(Stroke 18, p. 545, 1987; Ref. 2, pp. 282–285)*

57. **B.** In hypertensives, diabetics, Afro-Americans, and women, ticlopidine has been reported to be effective in preventing stroke recurrence. Aspirin has *not* been shown to be effective in women or to prevent recurrent stroke. Anticoagulants are effective only for cardiogenic cerebral embolism. For arteriolar disease, CEA is not effective; however, blood pressure reduction and antiplatelet medication are effective in preventing stroke recurrence. *(Ref. 2, p. 266)*

58. **B.** In hypertensive patients, this pattern would be consistent with cerebellar hemorrhage. Lack of pupillary, respiratory, eye movement abnormalities, and normal consciousness are *not* consistent with pontine hemorrhage. Headache and ataxia are not consistent with vestibular neuronitis. *(Ref. 2, pp. 285–288)*

59. **C.** Emergency noncontrast CT should demonstrate cerebellar hemorrhage. *(Ref. 2, pp. 285–288; Ref. 4, pp. 134–137)*

60. **D.** Cerebellar hematoma may cause edema and mass effect leading to brainstem compression and tonsillar herniation. Because of this potential risk, *emergency* hematoma evacuation should be performed. *(Ref. 2, pp. 285–288; Ref. 4, pp. 134–137)*

61. **A.** The cerebellar vermis controls trunk and leg movements, whereas the cerebellar hemispheres control the upper extremities. With vermal hematoma, gait is impaired with sparing of the upper extremities. With unilateral cerebellar lesion involving both vermis and hemisphere, there would be unilateral ataxic syndrome involving the ipsilateral arm and leg. *(Ref. 1, pp. 971–973)*

62. **A.** This constellation of symptoms represents Cushing reflex (arterial hypertension, bradycardia, slowed respiration). It is caused by a posterior fossa mass, e.g., hematoma, which results in tonsillar herniation and subsequent brainstem compression. The potential complication of tonsillar herniation is the reason that surgical hematoma evacuation represents a neurosurgical *emergency*. *(Ref. 1, p. 315; Ref. 2, pp. 360 and 366)*

63. **A.** These symptoms are due to secondary medullary compression by the cerebellar tonsils. *(Ref. 1, p. 317; Ref. 2, pp. 360 and 366)*

64. **E.** This represents an emergency, and all efforts must be made to reverse the effects of herniation by removing the mass effect of the cerebellar hematoma. *(Ref. 2, p. 317)*

65. **A.** Aphasia and homonymous hemianopsia suggest left temporal lobe dysfunction. *(Ref. 1, pp. 8–11; Ref. 2, pp. 421–423)*

66. **B.** The sudden onset is consistent with a vascular mechanism. In herpes simplex encephalitis, there would be fever and prodromal signs. With temporal lobe glioma, onset would

also be more gradual and the course would be progressive deterioration. *(Ref. 4, pp. 8–11)*

67. **A.** CT would be the initial diagnostic study to demonstrate hemorrhage. *(Ref. 4, pp. 134–7)*

68. **D.** Angiogram should be performed to delineate possible etiologies of hemorrhage in a young, *normotensive* patient. The most common vascular abnormality would be arterio-venous malformation. *(Ref. 4, pp. 134–137)*

69. **C.** Vascular malformation (arteriovenous, cavernous, telangiectasia) would be the most likely etiology. An aneurysm bleeds primarily into subarachnoid, not intracerebral space. Amyloid causes brain hemorrhage in elderly (not young) patients. Full evaluation for coagulopathy, neoplasm, or systemic illness would be warranted in a young, normotensive patient with brain hemorrhage. *(Ref. 4, pp. 150–151)*

70. **A.** In a neurologically asymptomatic patient with carotid bruit, noninvasive study such as carotid Doppler duplex study should be performed to determine if there is carotid stenosis. *(Ref. 2, pp. 257–258; Ref. 4, pp. 116–118)*

71. **B.** Bruit indicates that flow is *turbulent* (not laminar). It does *not* necessarily indicate that there is *stenosis*. *(Ref. 2, pp. 257–258; Ref. 4, pp. 116–118)*

72. **A.** Based on results of ACAS, CEA should be performed if an asymptomatic patient has greater than 60% carotid stenosis. *(Journal of the American Medical Association 273, p. 1421, 1995)*

73. **A.** In hypertensive patients, MRI may show enlarged perivascular spaces; but these do not necessarily indicate occurrence of lacunar infarct. If located in subcortical gray matter, they do not indicate multiple sclerosis. The basal ganglia is not an arterial border zone and therefore border-zone infarctions do not occur in this region. *(Ref. 5, pp. 435–458)*

74. **A.** For CEA to be beneficial in relative stroke reduction, risk of surgical complication should be less than 3%. *(Journal of the American Medical Association 273, p. 1421, 1995)*

7

SEIZURES AND EPILEPSY

True or False

1. _____ Syncope is usually caused by neurological illness, and the most common etiologies are stroke and epilepsy.

2. _____ Partial complex seizures (PCS) are usually but not always caused by temporal lobe dysfunction and should initially be treated with Tegretol.

3. _____ Most patients diagnosed with epilepsy require treatment with at least two antiepileptic drugs (AED), and treatment should be continued for 2 years after the patient becomes seizure free.

4. _____ In patients with partial complex seizures, PET scan shows reduced metabolism in the temporal lobe in the interictal period and increased metabolism in the ictal state.

5. _____ In patients with petit mal seizures, EEG shows an 8-cps spike and slow wave discharge pattern which is maximally present during sleep.

6. _____ Drug intoxication is a common cause of seizures and must be excluded prior to initiating anti-epileptic drugs.

Multiple Choice

Choose the most correct response.

7. _____ This percentage of the population experiences at least one seizure during life:

    A. 1%
    B. 5%
    C. 10%
    D. 20%
    E. 25%

8. _____ New AED (gabapentin, lamotrigine, felbamate) share this effect:

    A. Do not induce the hepatic cytochrome P-450 enzyme system and do not interfere with oral contraceptive hormone metabolism
    B. No AED interactions
    C. Effective for absence seizures

    D. Long half-life
    E. No serious systemic toxicity

9. _____ The following AED are associated with oral contraceptive failures:

    A. Carbamazepine
    B. Phenytoin
    C. Phenobarbital
    D. Primidone
    E. All of the above

10. _____ The following is true of felbamate:

    A. No serious side effects
    B. Effective in Lennox-Gastaut syndrome
    C. Affects calcium channels
    D. No known AED interaction
    E. All of the above

11. _____ The following is true of lamotrigine:

    A. Mechanism of action is similar to that of phenytoin and carbamazepine
    B. Inhibits sodium channels
    C. Drugs that induce drug-metabolizing enzymes in liver decrease the half-life of lamotrigine
    D. Skin rash is a common side effect
    E. All of the above

12. _____ This percentage of patients continue to have seizures despite adequate therapy with single or multiple AED:

    A. 5%
    B. 15%
    C. 30%
    D. 50%
    E. 70%

13. _____ The following is true of gabapentin:

    A. Short half-life requires multiple dosing schedule
    B. Excreted unchanged by kidneys
    C. Drug cleared by dialysis
    D. May enhance release and activity of gamma-aminobutyric acid
    E. All of the above

14. _____ These features have been reported with psychogenic seizures:

A. Plantar extensor (Babinski) response
B. Autonomic changes
C. Urinary or fecal incontinence
D. None of the above
E. All of the above

15. _____ Potential side effects of Valproic acid include:

A. Gingival hyperplasia
B. Renal dysfunction
C. Tremor
D. Megaloblastic anemia
E. Systemic lupus erythematosus

16. _____ The difference between simple and complex partial seizure involves which of the following:

A. Level of consciousness
B. Bilateral versus unilateral movements
C. Presence of aura
D. EEG pattern
E. Response to medication

17. _____ Antiepileptic drugs utilized for partial complex seizures include:

A. Tegretol
B. Phenytoin
C. Lamictal
D. Phenobarbital
E. All of the above

18. _____ This antiepileptic drug has the least medication interaction:

A. Neurontin
B. Tegretol
C. Depakote
D. Phenytoin
E. Phenobarbital

19. _____ The combination of medications most likely to cause respiratory depression in treating status epilepticus is:

A. Valium and phenobarbital
B. Dilantin and phenobarbital
C. Ativan and Dilantin
D. Paraldehyde and Dilantin
E. Valium and Dilantin

20. _____ Which patient needs CT scan most urgently?

A. New-onset partial seizures
B. New-onset absence seizures
C. Recurrent status epilepticus
D. New-onset generalized seizures with fever in an alert 9-month-old infant
E. Petit mal seizures

21. _____ Side effects of phenytoin include:

A. Hirsutism
B. Gingival hyperplasia
C. Peripheral neuropathy
D. Lymphadenopathy-simulating lymphoma
E. All of the above

22. _____ The following is true of febrile seizures:

A. They develop initially between 6 months and 6 years of age
B. Each episode lasts less than 20 min
C. Generalized in type; may be treated with rectal diazepam if seizure is prolonged
D. Seizures occur on ascending limb of fever curve
E. All of the above

23. _____ Partial seizures include the following patterns:

A. Jacksonian march
B. Petit mal
C. Myoclonus
D. Syncope
E. Migraine

24. _____ The following EEG pattern is characteristic of a specific clinical seizure type:

A. Spike
B. Polyspike and wave
C. Spike and wave
D. None of the above
E. All of the above

25. _____ Normal EEG pattern and appropriate frequency are:

A. Alpha, 8–13 cps
B. Beta, >13 cps
C. Theta, 4–7 cps
D. All of the above
E. None of the above

26. _____ During convulsive status epilepticus, the following changes occur:

A. Initially, blood flow meets or exceeds brain metabolic requirements
B. With repeated seizures, blood flow diminishes such that it is not sufficient to meet brain metabolic demands

C. Initially, blood pressure is hypertensive; with repeated seizures, blood pressure may be low (hypotensive)
D. All of the above
E. None of the above

27. _____ The drug of choice for neonatal seizures is:

A. Diazepam
B. Phenobarbital
C. Depakote
D. Carbamazepine
E. Felbamate

28. _____ Medical complications of convulsive status epilepticus include:

A. Lactic acidosis, acute tubular necrosis
B. Cardiac arrhythmias
C. Pulmonary edema
D. Hyperpyrexia
E. All of the above

From the clinical history, choose the most appropriate response.

A 6-year-old boy is inattentive and day-dreaming in school. He appears to be a "behavior problem" because he does not pay attention. EEG shows 3-cps spike-and-wave activity during hyperventilation.

29. _____ The most likely diagnosis is:

A. Absence seizures
B. Partial complex seizures
C. Hyperactivity—attention deficit disorder
D. Narcolepsy
E. Cataplexy

30. _____ Appropriate treatment would be:

A. Depakote
B. Tegretol
C. Ritalin
D. Elavil
E. Inderal

31. _____ Further diagnostic studies should include:

A. Sphenoidal EEG
B. Polysomnogram
C. CT
D. MRI
E. None of the above

32. _____ Todd's paralysis is associated with:

A. Permanent hemiplegia
B. Transient aphasia
C. Epileptiform discharges
D. Flat-line EEG
E. Hyponatremia

J.R. is an 18-year-old college freshman. While studying for final examinations, he is observed to have a single generalized major motor seizure. He is brought to the Emergency Department and is found to be neurologically normal.

33. _____ The initial diagnostic study should be:

A. Urine toxicology
B. CT
C. MRI
D. EEG
E. LP

34. _____ If all diagnostic tests are normal, management should be:

A. Initiate phenobarbital
B. Initiate phenytoin
C. Admit to hospital for video monitoring
D. Begin ketogenic diet
E. Utilize no antiepileptic medication; observe to determine if further episodes occur. Caution to avoid sleep deprivation.

A 32-year-old woman has multiple "epileptic attacks" despite adequate blood levels of phenytoin and carbamazepine. These attacks always occur at work and are precipitated by stressful episodes. She feels "drugged" on this level of medication and has suffered three serious falls due to disequilibrium. EEG is normal on three occasions.

35. _____ Management should include:

A. Increase dose of current AED
B. Add another AED
C. Discontinue current AED and substitute Depakote
D. Video monitoring of the patient
E. Discontinue current AED and begin psychotherapy for "psychogenic seizures"

36. _____ Diagnostic studies should include:

A. MRI
B. CT
C. LP
D. Obtain serum prolactin within 30 min of next attack
E. Polysomnogram

P.T. is a 15-year-old adolescent who develops myoclonic jerks involving the arms upon awakening. Two months later she has a generalized convulsion.

37. _____ The most likely diagnosis is:

   A. Juvenile myoclonic epilepsy
   B. Syncope
   C. Partial complex seizures
   D. Complex absence seizures
   E. Psychogenic seizures

38. _____ If AED were utilized and she became seizure free, criteria to discontinue AED would include:

   A. Normal examination
   B. Normal EEG
   C. Normal CT/MRI
   D. Seizure free for 24 months
   E. All of the above

A 35-year-old woman has episodes of "seizures" in which she has an aura of intense fear followed by loss of awareness with out-of-phase pelvic thrusting activity, urinary incontinence, and tongue biting, but no postictal confusion. EEG shows nonspecific slowing. She has therapeutic levels of Tegretol and Dilantin but continues to have daily seizures.

39. _____ Suggestions for management would include:

   A. Increase antiepileptic dose
   B. Switch to alternative antiepileptic medication
   C. Abruptly discontinue antiepileptic medication
   D. Consider epileptic surgery
   E. Perform video monitoring

40. _____ Diagnostic possibilities include:

   A. Partial complex seizures
   B. Frontal lobe seizures
   C. Supplementary motor cortex seizures
   D. Psychogenic nonepileptic seizures
   E. All of the above

41. _____ Important psychiatric factors which might be important in assessing the possible seizure type include:

   A. Sexual abuse
   B. Abandonment
   C. Hallucinations
   D. Delusions
   E. None of the above

42. _____ Following an episode, this test may be diagnostically useful:

   A. Serum prolactin
   B. CPK
   C. Serum sodium
   D. CT
   E. MRI

43. _____ Clinical features which suggest psychogenic non-epileptic seizures include:

   A. Bilateral motor signs with normal level of consciousness
   B. Absence of stereotypic seizure pattern
   C. Inducible or suggestible seizures
   D. Side-to-side motor movements
   E. All of the above

44. _____ With psychogenic nonepileptic seizures, EEG may show:

   A. Myogenic artifacts which may simulate epileptic discharge
   B. 14 and 6 positive bursts
   C. Wicket waves
   D. All of the above
   E. None of the above

A 10-year-old boy has a nocturnal generalized seizure. Following the episode, he is confused, afebrile, but has no other neurological abnormality. EEG shows bilateral centrotemporal spikes. No AED is initiated until he has a second nocturnal seizure 8 months later.

45. _____ The most likely diagnosis is:

   A. Sleep myoclonus
   B. Absence seizures
   C. Rolandic epilepsy
   D. Partial complex seizures
   E. All of the above

46. _____ The next diagnostic study should be:

   A. CT
   B. MRI
   C. Skull radiogram
   D. LP
   E. None of the above

47. _____ Treatment should be:

   A. Valproic acid
   B. Phenytoin
   C. Phenobarbital
   D. Primidone
   E. No AED warranted

RESPONSES AND EXPLANATIONS

1. F. Syncope is characterized by brief loss of consciousness and loss of postural tone, followed by immediate and complete recovery. It is caused by transient reversible decrease in cerebral blood flow. Syncope is almost *never* caused by neurological illness but is most commonly due to systemic factors. Potentially serious cardiac disease *must* be excluded in syncope patients. *(Ref. 1, pp. 12–19; Ref. 2, pp. 207–209)*

2. T. PCS usually are due to mesial temporal lobe dysfunction but may originate from other regions, most commonly the frontal lobe. At onset, consciousness is impaired. Many AED are effective (phenytoin, phenobarbital, valproate, mysoline), but carbamazepine is the drug of choice. *(Ref. 2, pp. 332–334, 341–342; Ref. 4, pp. 168–169)*

3. F. At least 60% of patients are controlled with monotherapy with low incidence of side effects. When a second drug is added (polytherapy), there is a slight increase to 70% of patients controlled; however, there is a marked increase of drug-induced side effects due to polypharmacy. If the patient is seizure free for 2 years, has normal examination, and EEG and CT/MRI are normal, consider discontinuing AED; however, if this is done, 25% of patients will have seizure recurrence. *(Annals of Internal Medicine 120, pp. 411–422, 1994; New England Journal of Medicine 308, pp. 1508–1515, 1576–1590, 1981; New England Journal of Medicine 323, pp. 1468–1476, 1990)*

4. T. During the interictal state, metabolism in the abnormal temporal lobe tissue is reduced; during a seizure episode, however, there is increased cerebral blood flow and metabolism in the pathological temporal lobe. *(Ref. 2, pp. 310, 313, 318)*

5. F. EEG shows 3-cps spike-and-wave symmetrical discharges. These are best seen following hyperventilation. In other seizure types, seizure may be precipitated by sleep deprivation. *(Ref. 4, pp. 164–165)*

6. T. In patients who present with a single seizure, perform drug toxicology. Many drugs (alcohol, antihistamines, sympathomimetics, antidepressants) may cause seizures. Many illicit drugs, including cocaine, phencyclidine (PCP), T's and blues (Talwin and Pyribenzamine), may cause seizures. Remember that withdrawal of certain CNS depressant medication may also cause seizures (barbiturates, diazepam). For example, long-term use of Fiorinal (for headache), which contains barbiturate, may cause seizure following abrupt withdrawal. *(Neurologic Clinics of North America 12, pp. 85–100, 1994; Ref. 4, pp. 160–161)*

7. B. Patients may have a single unprovoked seizure or febrile seizure. Therefore not all first or single seizures need to be treated. A single seizure does not define epilepsy, which is defined as *recurrent* unprovoked seizures. *(Ref. 4, pp. 160–161)*

8. A. The only *common* factor is no effect on oral contraceptive metabolism. Gabapentin does not interact with other AED and is excreted unchanged in the urine. The other AED have significant interactions and effects on hepatic metabolism. Felbamate has serious systemic toxicity (especially aplastic anemia), and this limits its use. None of these AED is effective for absence seizures. *(Neurologic Clinics of North America 11, pp. 905–950, 1993; Neurology 46, pp. 1534–1539, 1996)*

9. E. Enzyme-inducing AED may reduce oral contraceptive (OCP) estradiol levels by 40% and may reduce free progestin levels. They may *increase* OCP failures. Nonhepatic enzyme-inducing AED—Valproic acid and gabapentin—do not have this effect. *(Neurology 46, pp. 1534–1539, 1996)*

10. B. After felbamate was FDA approved, aplastic anemia and hepatic toxicity were reported. If it is utilized, weekly or biweekly complete blood count and liver function tests are recommended. Felbamate affects sodium channels. Valproic acid decreases Felbamate clearance; phenytoin and carbamazepine increase clearance of Felbamate. Felbamate is *very* effective in Lennox-Gastaut syndrome. *(Ref. 2, p. 325)*

11. E. Lamotrigine is an effective AED for partial and secondary generalized seizures. Valproic acid slows lamotrigine metabolism, whereas other AED decrease the half-life of lamotrigine. Skin rash is most common if lamotrigine is used with Valproic acid. Other side effects include headache, dizziness, diplopia, tremor, and GI discomfort. *(Ref. 2, pp. 324–325)*

12. C. Approximately 25–30% of epileptic patients continue to have seizures. Approximately 60% of patients are controlled with monotherapy, and an additional 10–15% are controlled with polypharmacy. With polypharmacy, the incidence of side effects increases from approximately 15% (with monotherapy) to 50%. *(Annals of Internal Medicine 120, pp. 411–422, 1994)*

13. E. All are true. This AED has few side-effects—somnolence, fatigue, ataxia, and GI discomfort. It has no interactions with other AED. It is effective for partial and secondary generalized seizures. *(Ref. 2, pp. 324–325)*

14. E. All listed features may occur in psychogenic seizures. Although positive Babinski sign has been *reported* in psychogenic seizures, this author believes that their occurrence is *very* strong evidence that the patient experienced an *epileptic* seizure. These features are *usually* considered definite evidence of epileptic seizures; however, based on video-monitoring experience, we know that incontinence and autonomic features can occur with psychogenic seizures. Their occurrence in psychogenic seizures emphasizes the difficulty of differentiating psychogenic from epileptic seizures based on clinical features alone. It is crucial to have normal EEG observed during an episode to be certain that the episode represents psychogenic seizure. *(Neurology 46, pp. 1499–1506, 1996)*

15. **C.** Valproic acid has major systemic toxicity—liver dysfunction. This occurs most commonly in children less than 2 years old and in patients who utilize multiple AED. Of neurological toxicities, postural and intentional tremor are most common. *(Ref. 2, pp. 322–323)*

16. **A.** In patients with partial (focal) seizures, the level of consciousness or awareness is initially impaired in *complex* partial seizures, e.g., psychomotor or temporal lobe seizures, whereas consciousness is normal in *simple* partial seizures, e.g., Jacksonian motor seizures. Aura occurs in partial seizures, but does *not* occur in generalized seizures. EEG shows focal pattern in partial seizures; however, routine surface EEG may need to be supplemented by nasopharyngeal, sphenoidal, or even depth electrodes (done only as part of surgical epilepsy evaluation) to demonstrate focal EEG discharge. *(Ref. 4, pp. 166–170)*

17. **E.** All listed drugs are effective for control of partial complex seizures. Phenobarbital is less well tolerated because of its potential effect on cognitive function, whereas carbamazepine and phenytoin have more systemic toxicity. Lamictal is newly approved for seizures, especially partial complex seizures, but this AED has a high incidence of skin rash. *(Ref. 2, pp. 322–323; Ref. 4, pp. 166–170)*

18. **A.** Gabapentin (Neurontin) does not interact or influence blood levels of other AED. This makes it a unique AED, as all other drugs have potential interactions which may raise or lower the levels of other AED. *(Ref. 2, pp. 321–325)*

19. **A.** Status epilepticus represents continuous seizures, from which the patient fails to regain consciousness between attacks. There is a potential risk of permanent neuronal injury resulting from hypoxic-ischemic brain damage, hyperthermia, lactic acidosis, hypoglycemia, cardiac arrhythmias, and respiratory depression. Initial management includes ventilatory and cardiovascular support. Treat with *intravenous* AED. Combined use of diazepam and phenobarbital is potentially dangerous due to synergistic hypotension and respiratory depression. In addition, diazepam has potential for cardiac toxicity. *(Ref. 2, pp. 343–346; Ref. 4, pp. 176–177)*

20. **A.** Partial seizures are due to underlying structural brain disease, which may be micro- or macroscopic. Absence or petit mal seizures are generalized in type, and it is unlikely that structural (focal) lesion will be demonstrated by CT/MRI. Seizures occurring in a febrile infant probably represent febrile seizures and not meningitis. In this case, LP would be warranted prior to CT in evaluating the *initial* febrile seizure. Recurrent status epilepticus would probably be due to noncompliance with AED regimen or less possibly an underlying structural lesion. *(Ref. 2, pp. 331–335)*

21. **E.** Cosmetic side effects which lead to noncompliance with phenytoin include hirsutism and gingival hyperplasia. Peripheral neuropathy occurs with *long-term* phenytoin utilization. Lymph node enlargement which may *simulate* lymphoma occurs but is *usually* reversible when phenytoin is discontinued. *(Ref. 2, pp. 322–323)*

22. **E.** These consist of brief episodes of generalized major motor seizures. They frequently occur in patients who have positive family history of this seizure type. Recurrence after initial febrile seizure occurs in one-third of patients. After the *initial* seizure, it is important to exclude CNS infection. Treatment with AED has not been shown to prevent development of epilepsy. *(Ref. 2, pp. 338, 391)*

23. **A.** Partial seizures indicate focal unilateral activation of a specific anatomical cerebral cortical region, e.g., motor, somatosensory, visual, auditory. Jacksonian seizures usually begin with clonic rhythmical flexion thumb movements that spread to adjacent muscle groups—wrist, arm, shoulder—and later spread to either the leg or face. Myoclonic and petit mal are generalized seizures. *(Ref. 4, pp. 164–165, 166–8)*

24. **D.** In patients with epilepsy, there is excessive and paroxysmal neural discharges (cerebral dysrhythmia). This may be manifested by sharp waves, spikes, or rhythmical slow waves. These may be seen in any type of epilepsy. Only in absence seizures is there characteristic 3-cps spike and slow wave pattern. *(Neurologic Clinics of North America 11, pp. 857–883, 1993)*

25. **D.** The basic symmetrical background frequency is 8–13 cps. This is maximal in the occipital region and is referred to as *alpha* rhythm. In the frontal region, there may be more rapid and lower-amplitude *beta* (14–30 cps) activity. There may be intermittent infrequent *theta* (3–7 cps) in normals, but if this slow wave pattern is more frequent than the alpha rhythm, this is abnormal. *(Ref. 2, pp. 48–51)*

26. **D.** With clinical seizures, blood flow increases to meet increased metabolic demands of the brain. However, with repeated seizures, the patient becomes hypotensive, hypoxic, lactic acidotic, and hypoglycemic, and these effects may cause permanent neuronal damage. In the early phase of status epilepticus, sympathetic changes may result in hypertension and tachycardia, but later hypotension develops. Due to intense muscle contraction which occurs with repeated seizures, muscle breakdown and rhabdomyolysis may occur. *(Ref. 2, pp. 343–346; Ref. 4, pp. 176–177)*

27. **B.** Neonatal seizures may consist of tonic head or neck deviation, oral-buccal movements, opisthotonic posturing, or myoclonic movements. They may be confused with normal jitteriness or myoclonus of sleep. Treatment consists of phenobarbital or phenytoin. If seizures do not respond to AED, *pyridoxine* deficiency should be suspected as well as other metabolic disturbances (hypoglycemia, hypomagnesemia, hypocalcemia). *(Neurologic Clinics of North America 11, pp. 755–776, 1993)*

28. **E.** Mortality from status epilepticus is 25%. Outcome is best in patients with known epilepsy who have abruptly discontinued their anticonvulsants and worse in cases in which there is an underlying brain lesion, e.g., hypoxia-ischemia, brain hemorrhage. Neurogenic pulmonary edema and cardiac arrhythmias may develop. Rhabdomyolysis and myoglobinuria may lead to acute renal failure. Intense muscle contraction and autonomic discharge may lead to hyperpyrexia. *(Ref. 2, pp. 343–346; Ref. 4, pp. 176–177)*

29. **A.** Absence seizures occur without prodrome or aura. The patient appears unresponsive, as if not paying attention. There is no associated motor activity as contrasted to the automatisms of partial complex seizures. In cataplexy, there is sudden loss of muscle tone due to emotional stimulus. In narcolepsy, the patient appears to sleep; however, EEG does not show spike-and-wave pattern. *(Ref. 2, pp. 164–165)*

30. **A.** Valproic acid (Depakane) or divalproex sodium (Depakote) is the most appropriate treatment. Since some patients later develop major motor seizures, this AED has broad spectrum for seizure control and may be effective for preventing this occurrence. Ethosuximide (Zarontin) is effective *only* for absence seizures. Tegretol is used for partial seizures and *not* for absence seizures. The other listed drugs have no AED potential. *(Ref. 2, pp. 164–165)*

31. **E.** For patients with generalized seizures, CT or MRI are not necessary. For possible partial complex seizures, nasopharyngeal or sphenoidal electrodes are helpful to demonstrate temporal lobe spikes which may not be seen with routine EEG montages. A polysomnogram would be useful if narcolepsy is suspected. *(Ref. 2, pp. 160–161)*

32. **B.** Todd postictal paralysis may develop following seizures, as seizures may induce reversible alterations in neuronal function. The effect is most commonly paralysis but may be aphasia, visual, or sensory defect. Duration is usually less than 24 hr but may be several days. Permanent deficit does *not* occur. The mechanism is probably neuronal hyperpolarization reflecting enhanced CNS inhibition. *(Ref. 2, pp. 310, 313,318)*

33. **A.** In younger patients with a single seizure, consider the possibility that it is drug induced. Over-the-counter medications utilized to enhance alertness and attention, cold remedies, and diet pills may lower the seizure threshold. Prior to

initiating full neurodiagnostic evaluation, it is important to know if any drug was ingested. Incidence of a single seizure is 9%, but only 3% will develop epilepsy; therefore only one-third of patients who have a single seizure will have recurrence. *(Annals of Internal Medicine 120, pp. 411–422, 1994; Ref. 2, p. 349)*

34. **E.** If all studies are negative, there is no family history of epilepsy, and there is a precipitating factor—e.g., emotional stress, sleep deprivation, precipitating drug history—it is not clear whether AED should be initiated. There is a 34–71% recurrence rate after a single seizure in adults. If EEG is normal, the recurrence rate is less than 25%. Recurrence usually occurs within 24 months. If AED are utilized and the patient is seizure free, discontinuation can be considered. If *no* AED are utilized for the first seizure, certain restrictions in driving and potentially dangerous activities should be mandated. *(Ref. 2, pp. 160–161)*

35. **D.** Most patients respond to appropriate AED, especially when therapeutic blood levels indicate compliance. If multiple AED are utilized, this causes increasing problems with drug interactions. Prior to switching medications, it is important to determine if these attacks may represent *nonepileptic attacks*. This is best done by observing an episode with video-EEG monitoring. *(Neurology 46, pp. 1499–1506, 1996)*

36. **D.** If an attack is observed, obtain serum prolactin within 30 min. Serum prolactin is elevated in partial complex seizures and generalized major motor attacks but shows no elevation following psychogenic (nonepileptic) seizure. Regardless of serum prolactin level, perform video monitoring. Carefully question the patient for prior history of physical or sexual abuse if a psychogenic seizure is suspected. *(Neurology 46, pp. 1499–1506, 1996)*

37. **A.** Juvenile myoclonic epilepsy has its onset in the teenage years. It consists of myoclonus, absence, and generalized major motor seizures. Myoclonus occurs in the morning and involves the upper extremities. These seizures respond to Valproic acid but *not* to phenytoin or carbamazepine. *(Ref. 2, p. 338)*

38. **E.** All the listed criteria are appropriate and should be present prior to deciding to discontinue AED. Remember that certain seizures are age-specific, e.g., absence seizures. These patients mature to being at low risk of seizure recurrence; however, if recurrence occurs in an adult patient, changes in lifestyle may be mandated (loss of driving privilege, job loss, recreational restrictions). If AED medication is stopped, *very* gradual withdrawal (over many months) is necessary to reduce risk of seizure recurrence. *(Ref. 4, pp. 162–163)*

39. **E.** This is a very difficult case which has some features suggesting both epileptic and nonepileptic seizures. EEG is not normal but shows no epileptiform discharges. Be cognizant

that 5–10% of the normal population has nonspecific abnormalities, or muscle artifact (due to patient movement) may be present that simulate spikes. In this difficult case, video monitoring should be performed before making management decisions. *(Ref. 2, pp. 339–343; Ref. 4, pp. 170–171)*

40. **E.** Partial complex seizures may originate from the temporal or frontal lobes. Supplementary motor cortex seizures may simulate psychogenic seizures. *(Ref. 4, pp. 168–169)*

41. **A.** If the patient had a prior history of physical or sexual abuse, this would make the clinician sensitive to the possibility of psychogenic seizure; however, clinical factors must be evaluated independently. Remember that patients with psychogenic seizures may also have epileptic seizures. *(Ref. 4, pp. 170–171)*

42. **A.** Following an episode of partial complex or major motor seizures, serum prolactin is frequently elevated. Following generalized but not usually partial complex seizure, CPK is usually elevated due to intense muscle contractions. *(Ref. 4, pp. 170–171)*

43. **E.** With psychogenic seizures, all listed features are present. With bilateral motor activity due to epileptic seizure, it would be expected that consciousness would be impaired. In epileptic seizures, the seizure pattern is repetitive and stereotyped. If seizures always occur when observers are present or if attacks are easily inducible, consider psychogenic seizures. *(Neurology 46, pp. 1499–1506, 1996)*

44. **D.** When a patient has a seizure of any type, muscle artifact may occur which simulates spike activity on EEG. Also, certain nonspecific EEG abnormalities are not indicative of cerebral dysrhythmia. *(Ref. 2, pp. 49–53)*

45. **C.** Benign childhood epilepsy with centrotemporal spikes (Rolandic epilepsy) has onset between ages 3 and 13. Seizures begin as simple partial, usually involving the face and then may secondarily generalize. Seizures invariably occur at night. *(Ref. 2, pp. 392–393)*

46. **E.** EEG findings are characteristic, consisting of high-amplitude spikes and sharp waves in the central region—most frequently observed during light sleep. This frequently results from a genetic disorder with an autosomal dominant pattern. If all features are characteristic, further neurodiagnostic studies are usually unnecessary. *(Ref. 2, pp. 392–393)*

47. **B.** Patients with Rolandic epilepsy usually stop having seizures by age 15; therefore, AED can be safely discontinued after this time. These seizures are usually easily controlled with phenytoin or carbamazepine. *(Ref. 2, pp. 392–393)*

8

SYNCOPE, VERTIGO, DIZZINESS

True or False

1. _____ Vertigo is the delusion or illusion of movement experienced by a patient, in which the body or the environment is moving.

2. _____ In patients who are experiencing true vertigo, nystagmus should be present on clinical examination when the patient is vertiginous.

3. _____ Vertigo may be caused by disturbances in the peripheral or central vestibular pathways.

4. _____ In patients with vertical nystagmus due to peripheral etiology, other brainstem or cerebellar findings are observed on the neurological examination.

5. _____ Ataxia, dysmetria, and incoordination are usually associated with a resting tremor.

6. _____ Disequilibrium or imbalance can be caused by cerebellar or posterior column disorders.

7. _____ The critical sensors of body orientation are the labyrinthine and visual systems.

8. _____ Epilepsy and migraine are common causes of vertigo.

9. _____ Isolated vertigo is a characteristic symptom of vertebrobasilar TIA.

10. _____ Syncope is a common clinical feature of supra- or infratentorial neurological disorders.

11. _____ In a patient with vertigo, vomiting and autonomic dysfunction (heart rate changes, diaphoresis) suggest brainstem lesions.

12. _____ In patients with suspected syncope, the occurrence of isolated myoclonic jerks and/or urinary incontinence should alert the physician to seizures as the more likely diagnosis.

13. _____ Patients with convulsive syncope should be treated with antiepileptic drugs.

14. _____ Following syncope, myalgias and headache are common complaints.

15. _____ During a syncopal episode, EEG shows either diffuse slowing or spike-and-wave activity.

Matching

Match the clinical features with the correct diagnosis.

A. Vertigo which develops when the patient turns over in bed

B. Vertigo, tinnitus, high-pitched hearing loss

C. Episodic vertigo, difficulty with speech discrimination, sensori-neural hearing loss

D. Sudden onset of vertigo and vomiting with normal hearing

E. Dizziness and light-headedness with acral paresthesias

16. _____ Psychogenic dizziness

17. _____ Benign positional vertigo (BPV)

18. _____ Meniere disease

19. _____ Acoustic neurinoma

20. _____ Viral labyrinthitis

Multiple Choice

Respond based on the clinic history.

M.M. is a 21-year-old female college student who has episodes of feeling dizzy and having her vision "gray out." After this she loses consciousness and falls limply to the floor. Immediately after recovering consciousness, she is neurologically normal. She has a strong family history of cardiovascular and cerebrovascular disease, smokes heavily, takes oral contraceptive medication, and was told of borderline hypertension 5 years ago. For the past 2 weeks she has been nauseated in the *morning*, and she vomited on one occasion.

21. _____ The most likely diagnosis is:

A. SAH
B. Ischemic stroke
C. Intracerebral hemorrhage
D. Seizure
E. Syncope

22. _____ The initial diagnostic test should be:

    A. CT
    B. MRI
    C. EEG
    D. EKG
    E. LP

23. _____ Other important diagnostic studies which might reveal the cause of the symptoms in this case include:

    A. Cortisol level
    B. 24-hr urine determination for 5-hydroxy-indole acetic acid
    C. Pregnancy test
    D. Antiphospholipid antibody test
    E. Catecholamine screen for pheochromocytoma

24. _____ Treatment for this condition might include this medication:

    A. Beta-blocking agent
    B. Calcium channel blocker
    C. Atropine
    D. Depakote
    E. None of the above

J.B. is a 50-year-old alcoholic who falls frequently. Examination shows truncal and gait ataxia; normal finger-to-nose but impaired heel-to-shin maneuver; normal reflexes, strength, and sensation. He has no family history of neurological disorders.

25. _____ Most likely etiology for this neurological condition is:

    A. Hypothyroidism
    B. Wilson's disease
    C. Paraneoplastic disorder
    D. Inherited cerebellar degeneration
    E. None of the above

26. _____ Pathology is most likely located in this brain region:

    A. Vermis of cerebellum
    B. Cerebellar hemispheres
    C. Brainstem
    D. Thalamus
    E. Substantia nigra

27. _____ Diagnostic studies would be warranted to exclude this condition:

    A. Wilson's disease
    B. Parkinson's disease
    C. Cerebellar neoplasm
    D. Peripheral neuropathy
    E. Cerebellar atrophy

28. _____ Effective treatment for the neurological disorder would be:

    A. Thiamine
    B. Pyridoxine
    C. B_{12}
    D. Thyroid hormone
    E. None of the above

A 22-year-old has an aura of light-headedness, weak and rubbery legs, and visual blurring. He falls to the ground and becomes rigid. He experiences multiple myoclonic jerks of his left arm, followed by a single myoclonic jerk of his right leg. He urinates on himself and bites his tongue. Immediately following this episode, he rapidly regains consciousness with no postepisode confusion.

29. _____ The most likely diagnosis is:

    A. Major motor seizure
    B. Psychogenic seizure
    C. Partial complex seizure
    D. Syncope
    E. Vertebro-basilar TIA

30. _____ A high-yield diagnostic test would be:

    A. LP
    B. EEG
    C. CT
    D. MRI
    E. Tilt-table test

31. _____ Treatment of neurocardiogenic syncope might include:

    A. Inderal
    B. Isuprel
    C. Nifedipine
    D. Phenytoin
    E. Imipramine

A 70-year-old woman has a 4-month history of intermittent whirling sensation of her body and head when she rolls over in bed. On examination, hanging-head maneuver elicits rotatory nystagmus with fast component to the left side. There is a latency of 3 sec before onset of nystagmus. Hearing is normal, and the remainder of the neurological examination is normal.

32. _____ The most likely diagnosis is:

    A. Wallenberg syndrome
    B. Benign positional vertigo (BPV)
    C. Multiple sclerosis
    D. Vestibular neuronitis
    E. Acoustic neuroma

33. _____ Cost-effective diagnostic studies include:

   A. CT
   B. MRI
   C. Brainstem evoked potentials
   D. Electronystagmography
   E. None of the above

34. _____ The most effective treatment would be:

   A. Vestibular suppressants
   B. Antiemetics
   C. Vestibular neurectomy
   D. Posterior fossa craniotomy
   E. Crystal particle repositioning maneuvers and vestibular exercises

RESPONSES AND EXPLANATIONS

1. **T.** Vertigo implies sensation of *motion* in either the horizontal or vertical plane. The patient reports moving relative to the environment or the environment moving relative to the patient. Vertigo is due to vestibular dysfunction. This may involve the peripheral labyrinth or the central vestibular pathway (including the flocculus of the cerebellum). *(Neurology 22, p. 323, 1972; Ref. 2, p. 120)*

2. **T.** Patients with vertigo due to vestibular dysfunction usually show nystagmus on clinical examination. The presence of nystagmus can be confirmed by electronystagmogram. *(The Neurologist 1, p. 125, 1995; Ref. 2, pp. 119–123)*

3. **T.** Vertigo can be caused by dysfunction in the peripheral or central vestibular pathways. It is most intense with *peripheral* disturbances. *(Ref. 1, pp. 30–35; Ref. 2, p. 125)*

4. **T.** With labyrinthine or peripheral vestibular disturbances, nystagmus is horizontal or rotational. Vertical nystagmus indicates brainstem dysfunction due to either structural lesion or medication effect, e.g., phenytoin toxicity. *(Ref. 2, pp. 133–134)*

5. **F.** Ataxia and incoordination are consistent with cerebellar dysfunction. Cerebellar tremor may be *postural* or intentional. *Resting* tremor indicates basal ganglia dysfunction. *(Ref. 2, pp. 147–150)*

6. **T.** Disequilibrium is a sensation of *imbalance* when the patient is walking or standing. It may be caused by multiple motor (parkinsonism, cerebellar, hydrocephalus) or sensory (proprioceptive impairment due to peripheral nerve or spinal cord) disturbances. *(Ref. 2, p. 120)*

7. **T.** The critical sensors of body orientation are the labyrinth and the visual system. Primary visual disorders may rarely cause dizziness. The sensory receptors in the labyrinth are the saccule and utricle. *(Ref. 2, pp. 121–122)*

8. **F.** Both conditions are extremely rare causes of dizziness and vertigo. With epileptic focus in the posterior temporal region, epileptic dizzy spells lasting only a few seconds may occur. In patients with "basilar" migraine, vertigo may occur with associated headache. It cannot be emphasized too strongly that these are *very* uncommon causes of vertigo. *(Ref. 2, p. 135)*

9. **F.** With vertebro-basilar TIA, *isolated* dizziness, disequilibrium, diplopia, dysarthria, and dysphagia are *most uncommon.* Characteristic features of this type of TIA are constellations of symptoms such as brief episode of vertigo, diplopia, ataxia, dysarthria, incoordination, *and* facial numbness which comes on *suddenly* and resolves completely in 20 min. Isolated symptoms are rarely TIA, whereas combinations of symptoms including dizziness-vertigo may represent TIA. *(Ref. 2, p. 134)*

10. **F.** Syncope is caused by reduction in cerebral blood flow such that inadequate oxygen and glucose are delivered to the brain. It is *almost never* caused by primary neurological disorder. *(Annals of Internal Medicine 112, p. 85, 1990; Annals of Internal Medicine 116, p. 358, 1992)*

11. **F.** Autonomic dysfunction in vertigo is due to involvement of the vagal nerve but does *not* indicate that there is a brainstem lesion. In patients who experience intense vertigo, nausea and vomiting invariably occur. *(Ref. 1, pp. 30–35; Ref. 2, p. 129)*

12. **F.** In patients who experience syncope, isolated myoclonic jerks frequently occur. If myoclonic jerks are rhythmical and sustained, consider epileptic seizure. *(Journal of the American Medical Association 237, p. 1372, 1977; Ref. 2, p. 217)*

13. **F.** Convulsive syncope refers to a *primary* syncopal disorder in which there may be certain "convulsive" clinical features: tonic phase, isolated myoclonic jerks, incontinence. EEG does *not* show epileptiform activity. This is syncope and not epilepsy; AED are not indicated as treatment, as the primary mechanism is syncope with prolonged cerebral ischemia. *(Annals of Neurology 11, p. 525, 1982; Ref. 2, pp. 217–218)*

14. **F.** Following seizure, myalgias occur due to intense muscle contractions. Headache due to cerebral vasodilation occurs with seizures. Neither of these symptoms occurs with syncope. *(Ref. 2, pp. 217–218)*

15. **F.** During a syncopal episode, there is a brief diffuse EEG slow-wave pattern which rapidly returns to normal immediately after the episode. Spike-and-wave activity is epileptogenic and would *not* occur with syncope. *(Ref. 2, pp. 216–218)*

16. **E.** Patients with emotional disorders may experience "dizziness." In hyperventilation and panic attacks, light-headedness with associated tingling around the mouth and extremities may occur. In unexplained dizziness, attempt to induce a typical attack by hyperventilating the patient for several minutes in an effort to induce characteristic symptoms. *(Ref. 2, pp. 136–137)*

17. **A.** Some patients experience vertigo *only* when they place their head in a certain position, e.g., turning over in bed. Symptoms of vertigo are associated with nystagmus on clinical examination. Symptoms can be reproduced by Nylen-Barany or Hallpike maneuver (place the patient on the examining

table and lower the head backwards until the head is 45 degrees below the edge of the table and then turn the patient to the right and then the left side). The goal of this maneuver is to reproduce the characteristic symptoms experienced by the patient. In BPV, this maneuver induces vertigo and nystagmus. *(Ref. 2, pp. 129–130)*

18. **B.** Meniere disease is due to abnormality of the membranous labyrinth. Symptoms include recurrent episodes of vertigo, tinnitus, and hearing loss. Caloric response is decreased on the involved side. Hearing loss occurs for low frequencies, with preserved speech (word) discrimination. With repeated episodes, hearing impairment usually progresses, and patient may become deaf. *(Ref. 2, pp. 131–132)*

19. **C.** With acoustic neuromas, vertigo is accompanied by hearing loss. Hearing tests demonstrate *retrococlear* hearing loss involving high-frequency tones, and there is impaired speech discrimination. Due to the proximity of the trigeminal, abducens, and facial nerves to the eighth nerve, they may be affected by acoustic neuroma, causing facial numbness and paresthesias, facial weakness, or horizontal diplopia. *(Ref. 2, pp. 133–134; Ref. 5, pp. 132–135)*

20. **D.** Acute vestibular neuronitis or labyrinthitis causes sudden onset of intense vertigo, nausea, imbalance, and motion sensitivity. Examination shows rotatory or horizontal nystagmus *only*. This disorder usually follows upper respiratory infection or is associated with inner ear infection. Symptoms are self-limited; they may last several days and then spontaneously resolve. *(Ref. 2, pp. 128–129)*

21. **E.** Syncope is the cause of 3% of emergency department visits. It is defined as sudden brief loss of consciousness and impaired postural tone with immediate complete recovery and no postepisode confusion. Based on the clinical features, differentiation of syncope from seizure or stroke should be easily accomplished. *(Ref. 2, pp. 207–210)*

22. **D.** Syncope is almost never caused by primary neurological disease. Syncope is usually a *benign* condition; however, serious underlying *cardiac disorders* must be excluded as the etiology. Sudden death can occur in 20–30% of patients due to cardiac etiology. If syncope occurs initially in middle-aged or elderly patients, evaluate carefully for cardiac disease. *(Ref. 2, pp. 207–210)*

23. **C.** Syncope can occur in the early stages of pregnancy for undetermined reasons and in the later stages due to the compressive effect of the fetus on venous return to the heart. Pheochromocytoma, Addison's disease, and carcinoid syndrome may be uncommon causes of syncope. *(Mayo Clinic Proceedings 70, p. 757, 1995; Ref. 2, pp. 219–221)*

24. **E.** Most cases of syncope are benign and require no treatment. Certainly, do not utilize AED, as syncope is not a symptom of epilepsy. Perform careful cardiac examination including Holter monitoring. Exclude endocrine-metabolic-hematological disorders. Perform *a tilt-table test* to attempt to induce syncope. If positive, this confirms the diagnosis of vasovagal (neurocardiogenic) syncope. This results from increased myocardial sympathetic C-fiber stimulation. C-fiber stimulation results in vagal activation which causes bradycardia, hypotension, and peripheral vasodilation. The C-fiber stimulation can be antagonized by beta-adrenergic receptor blocking agents. Despite hypotension and bradycardia being potential side effects of this medication, these agents are effective treatment. *(Ref. 2, pp. 219–223)*

25. **E.** Alcohol causes cerebellar vermis atrophy, resulting in gait and trunk instability. All the other listed disorders can cause cerebellar ataxia, but clinical features of this case are less consistent with other disorders. For example, with hypothyroidism, systemic manifestations should be prominent. With Wilson's disease, look for Kayser-Fleisher corneal ring. In paraneoplastic syndrome, there is *pancerebellar* disorder involving the trunk, legs, *and* arms. Lack of family history is inconsistent with inherited disorders. *(Ref. 1, pp. 690–693; Ref. 2, pp. 674–678)*

26. **A.** Alcohol causes cerebellar (midline) vermis atrophy and does not extend to involve the lateral cerebellar hemispheres. The clinical pattern of alcoholic cerebellar degeneration affects gait and trunk but spares the arms. *(Ref. 1, pp. 690–693; Ref. 2, pp. 674–675)*

27. **C.** CT/MRI is necessary to exclude cerebellar mass lesions. These may also confirm the presence of cerebellar atrophy. Serum ceruloplasmin should be performed to exclude Wilson's disease. There are no clinical findings to suggest neuropathy. *(Ref. 1, pp. 690–693)*

28. **E.** In malnourished alcoholics, multivitamins including thiamine and protein repletion should be initiated; however, cessation of alcohol intake is the most effective treatment. This is *not* Wernicke encephalopathy, so thiamine does not reverse the process. *(Ref. 2, pp. 477–478)*

29. **D.** This fits with a diagnosis of "convulsive" syncope. Syncope is the primary process; however, there are convulsive features. Myoclonus is *not* rhythmical or sustained. Incontinence may occur with either syncope (loss of bladder muscle tone) or seizure. Tongue biting may occur with syncope, but tongue *maceration* occurs only with seizure. *(Ref. 2, pp. 216–218)*

30. **E.** Because the clinical history is so consistent with syncope, EEG findings would be unlikely to change the clinical diagnosis. Neurodiagnostic studies are not necessary or indicated in syncope. A tilt-table test would be most useful to help confirm the diagnosis of neurocardiogenic syncope with convulsive features. *(Ref. 2, p. 218)*

31. **A.** Beta-adrenergic blocking agents which inhibit myocardial sympathetic C fibers would be appropriate treatment. *(Ref. 2, pp. 213–214)*

32. **B.** This is characteristic of BPV. The lack of other neurological or acoustic (hearing) abnormalities would exclude the other neurological or auditory conditions. To precipitate vertigo and nystagmus following performance of hanging head position maneuver clinically confirms the diagnosis of BPV. *(Ref. 2, pp. 130–131)*

33. **E.** With classic clinical features of peripheral labyrinthine disorder, CT/MRI would be unnecessary. If subclinical brainstem disorder is suspected, brainstem (auditory) evoked potentials would be indicated, e.g., multiple sclerosis; however, this is *not* indicated in this case. *(Ref. 2, pp. 128–130)*

34. **E.** This disorder is caused by loose otolith or calcified particles in the ampullae of the semicircular canals (capulolithiasis). By attempting to reposition these particles by vestibular exercises, this condition is effectively treated. Long-term use of vestibular suppressants is ineffective in managing BPV. *(Ref. 2, pp. 128–130)*

9

SLEEP STATES
AND SLEEP DISORDERS

True or False

1. _____ Many insomnia patients experience periodic nocturnal myoclonus, which may awaken them and exacerbate insomnia.

2. _____ Primary symptom of narcolepsy is excessive daytime sleepiness.

3. _____ Cataplexy is defined as physiological loss of muscle tone that develops as a response to an intense emotional state.

4. _____ Sleep-walking usually occurs during non-REM sleep.

Multiple Choice

Choose the most appropriate response.

5. _____ Which of these clinical features occur in narcolepsy?

   A. Cataplexy
   B. Hypnagogic hallucinations
   C. Disrupted night-time sleep patterns
   D. A and B only
   E. A, B, and C

6. _____ Sleep apnea may be associated with worsening of which of the following medical condition(s)?

   A. Hypertension
   B. Heart failure
   C. Arrhythmias
   D. All of the above
   E. None of the above

7. _____ Treatment of narcolepsy may include:

   A. CNS-stimulant medication
   B. REM-suppressing medication
   C. Antiepileptic medication
   D. A and B
   E. Electroconvulsive therapy

8. _____ This drug is most effective in treating cataplexy:

   A. Ritalin
   B. Tofranil
   C. Dexedrine
   D. Inderal
   E. Prozac

9. _____ A polysomnogram permits minute-to-minute analysis of the following physiological parameters:

   A. EEG sleep–wake stages
   B. Respiratory pattern
   C. Cardiac status
   D. Muscle tone
   E. All of the above

Matching

Match the statement with the appropriate sleep parameter.

   A. High level of ascending reticular activating system (ARAS) activity
   B. Reduced ARAS activity and involvement of pontine raphe nucleus
   C. Adrenergic nucleus ceruleus and cholinergic pontine tegmental field
   D. Lesion of serotonergic cells of raphe nucleus
   E. L-tryptophan

10. _____ Non-REM sleep

11. _____ REM sleep

12. _____ Awake state

13. _____ Natural sleep substance

14. _____ Insomnia

Match the features with the appropriate stage of sleep.

A. Hypotonus, rapid eye movements; EEG shows mixed frequency pattern
B. Slight hypotonus; patient may feel awake
C. Light sleep with predominant EEG pattern being theta; sleep spindles occur
D. Deep sleep with absent rapid eye movements; EEG shows prominent theta pattern
E. Deep sleep with EEG showing prominent delta pattern

15. _____ Stage I

16. _____ Stage II

17. _____ Stage III

18. _____ Stage IV

19. _____ Stage V

Match the clinical condition with the sleep disorder.

A. Excessive daytime sleepiness
B. Nocturnal walking episodes
C. Child develops panic state at night during stage III sleep
D. Frightening dreams develop during stage IV sleep
E. Muscle flaccidity develops in the morning upon awakening

20. _____ Sleep paralysis

21. _____ Nightmares

22. _____ Night terrors

23. _____ Narcolepsy

24. _____ Somnambulism

Multiple Choice

Respond based on the clinical history.

A 25-year-old obese, hoarse female has gained 120 lb over the last year and reports excessive daytime sleepiness. When examined, she falls asleep in the office and snores continuously. She is observed to have apnea during periods of sleep. Exam shows "frog-like" speech, increased facial hair, thinning of the lateral portion of the eyebrows, and "hung up" reflexes.

25. _____ What medical condition would you consider?

    A. Cushing syndrome
    B. Hypothyroidism
    C. Congestive heart failure
    D. All of the above
    E. None of the above

26. _____ What evaluation should be done?

    A. Polysomnogram
    B. Endocrine laboratory tests
    C. Chest radiogram
    D. All of the above
    E. None of the above

27. _____ What is the appropriate management strategy?

    A. Send to Weight Watchers for weight control
    B. Continuous positive airway pressure device
    C. High-dose Ritalin
    D. Sleep study to determine type and severity of sleep disorder
    E. Mestinon and Inderal treatment

A 21-year-old ectomorphic, histrionic female graduate student reports that she falls asleep frequently during the day. These episodes have occurred since she was age 17. Also, when she laughs, she falls to the ground but does not lose consciousness.

28. _____ What are the diagnostic possibilities?

    A. Atonic epilepsy
    B. Cataplexy
    C. Vertebral-basilar drop attack
    D. Gelastic epilepsy
    E. None of the above

29. _____ What is appropriate treatment for this disorder?

    A. Phenytoin
    B. Inderal
    C. Depakote
    D. Dexedrine and imipramine
    E. No treatment is indicated

30. _____ What symptoms are commonly associated with this condition?

    A. Hallucinations related to awakening from sleep and entering into sleep state
    B. Vasovagal syncope
    C. REM behavioral disorder
    D. Hypokalemic sleep paralysis
    E. Obstructive sleep apnea

A 400-lb man is referred for evaluation of confusional behavior and dream enactment during which he has punched, strangled, and kicked his wife. He claims amnesia for these episodes. He has no daytime abnormal behavioral episodes.

31. _____ Which are likely differential diagnostic possibilities?

    A. Psychiatric fugue state
    B. Sleep-walking
    C. Obstructive sleep apnea (OSA)
    D. REM behavior disorder
    E. All of the above

32. _____ Which diagnostic study would be most useful?

    A. Sleep-deprived EEG
    B. Polysomnogram
    C. Sleep EEG
    D. All of the above
    E. None of the above

33. _____ Treatment of this disorder includes:

    A. Clonazapam
    B. Diazepam
    C. Carbamazepine
    D. All of the above
    E. None of the above

RESPONSES AND EXPLANATIONS

1. **T.** Nocturnal myoclonus is characterized by repetitive, brief, lower-extremity jerking movements which occur during sleep. In restless leg syndrome, patients experience uncomfortable "crawling" sensation in the calves and thighs. This causes the patient to constantly move the feet to reduce uncomfortable sensations. Both conditions may occur in the same patient, and they may interfere with sleep to cause or exacerbate insomnia (defined as inability to initiate and maintain sleep). *(Neurologic Clinics of North America 14, p. 631, 1996)*

2. **T.** Narcolepsy causes excessive daytime sleepiness, occuring during work, driving, watching television. Episodes are likely to occur when the patient is relaxed. Narcoleptic patients go directly into REM sleep in less than 10 min when studied with polysomnogram or daytime multiple sleep latency test. *(Neurologic Clinics of North America 14, pp. 545–571, 1996; Ref. 2, pp. 742–745)*

3. **T.** Cataplexy is defined as pathologic loss of muscle tone that develops in response to intense emotional stimulus, e.g., laughing, crying. Cataplexy may cause the patient to fall to the ground or may consist of milder episodes in which the patient feels weak in the knees or feels that his or her jaw is drooping. Cataplexy occurs as part of the narcoleptic syndrome. *(Neurological Clinics of North America 14, pp. 548–549, 1996; Ref. 2, pp. 742–744)*

4. **T.** Somnambulism (sleep-walking) and sleep terrors occur during non-REM sleep. This disorder occurs in children and in the early part of sleep. The activity may be quite elaborate. It is important to differentiate sleep-walking from partial complex seizures. *(Neurological Clinics of North America 14, p. 679, 1996; Ref. 2, pp. 746–747)*

5. **D.** Narcolepsy (daytime sleep episodes) may include the following associated features:
   a. Cataplexy—loss of muscle tone in response to intense emotions, e.g., laughing, crying.
   b. Hypnagogic hallucinations—hallucinations which occur in the drowsy period.
   c. Sleep paralysis—loss of muscle tone which occurs upon awakening in the morning.
   (Ref. 2, pp. 742–745)

6. **D.** In patients with obstructive sleep apnea, there is a strain on the heart and increased intrathoracic pressure. This may cause the patient to become hypertensive or to develop pulmonary hypertension, cardiac arrhythmias, and cardiac failure. These potential complications are the strongest possible reason to treat this condition vigorously. *(Ref. 2, pp. 735–737, 740–742)*

7. **A.** Treatment of narcolepsy includes methylphenidate (Ritalin), and cataplexy responds to imipramine or protriptyline. *(Ref. 2, pp. 742–745)*

8. **B.** Tofranil (imipramine) is effective in treating cataplexy but is not effective for controlling narcolepsy. *(Ref. 2, pp. 742–744)*

9. **E.** A polysomnogram is more than simply an EEG taken at night. It provides important information about normal and abnormal sleep patterns and stages and, with the use of physiological sensors, it is possible to monitor cardiac, respiratory, and muscle tone abnormalities. For example, this procedure is ideal to monitor patients with suspected obstructive sleep apnea. *(Ref. 2, pp. 725–726)*

10. **B**
11. **C**
12. **A**
13. **E**
14. **D**

10–14. Wakefulness is maintained through high levels of ARAS and thalamic activity which stimulate cerebral cortex. With high levels of ARAS activity, sleep is not possible. Insomnia can be caused by lesions of the raphe nucleus and inhibition of serotonin synthesis. Sleep may be enhanced by L-tryptophan, which is a serotonin precursor. Non-REM sleep requires reduced ARAS activity and involvement of the serotoninergic system of the pontine raphe nuclei. For REM sleep, interaction between the adrenergic-producing cells of the nucleus ceruleus and the cholinergic pontine gigantocellular tegmental field is required. *(Ref. 6, pp. 260–264)*

15. **B**
16. **C**
17. **D**
18. **E**
19. **A**

15–19. Stage I represents the transition between wakefulness and sleep. The patient may feel awake, attention and thinking are slowed, muscle tone is slightly reduced, abnormal eye movements do not occur, EEG begins to slow. Stage II is the first definite sleep stage, and the patient looks asleep. Muscle tone is reduced and eye movements are absent, EEG shows slowing to theta pattern, sleep spindles and K-complexes occur. Stage III is the first of two deep sleep stages. Muscle tone is reduced and eye movements are absent. EEG shows theta in stage III and delta activity in stage IV. Stages I through IV represent non-REM sleep. Stage V is REM sleep. In REM sleep, hypotonus (reduced muscle tone) and rapid eye movements occur. EEG is similar to stage I, with a low-amplitude, mixed-frequency pattern. Active dreaming occurs during the REM sleep stage. *(Ref. 2, pp. 726–728)*

20. E
21. D
22. C
23. A
24. B

20–24. Sleep paralysis is part of the narcolepsy syndrome and is characterized by severe muscle weakness which occurs as the patient awakens. Nightmares occur during stage IV (REM sleep). These are differentiated as sleep or night terrors which are episodes in which the child cries out or screams, and exhibits panic. There are marked autonomic features associated with night terrors. Night terrors occur in stage III or IV sleep (non-REM sleep). They usually occur in children. Narcolepsy is defined as excessive daytime sleepiness. Somnambulism is parasomnia in which night-time walking occurs. *(Ref. 2, pp. 730, 742, 744, 747–748)*

25. B. It is important to keep in mind that patients with medical conditions may have sleep disturbances. Based on clinical history, disorders which would most likely cause this constellation are hypothyroidism or Cushing syndrome. The clinical findings favor hypothyroidism, especially with the reflex abnormality such that there is delayed relaxation phase. *(Neurological Clinics of North America 14, p. 622, 1996; Ref. 2, pp. 740–742)*

26. D. If the patient has untreated hypothyroidism as the cause of sleep disorder, this must be diagnosed and treated. In hypothyroidism, all body and organ functions are slowed. These patients develop right-sided congestive heart failure. Weight reduction will not be successful unless the underlying medical condition is corrected. A polysomnogram is needed to assess if there is obstructive sleep apnea and to assess potential cardiovascular and respiratory complications of OSA. These must be reversed while hypothyroidism and weight reduction are being corrected. *(Neurologic Clinics of North America 14, p. 597, 1996)*

27. B. While thyroid replacement therapy is being initiated, treatment with continuous positive airway pressure (CPAP) is necessary to reverse the nocturnal obstructive airway disturbance which is putting added strain on the cardiopulmonary system. CPAP acts like a physical splint to open the airway, and it also enhances tone in the oropharynx. With weight reduction, sleep mechanics will be improved to reduce apneic spells. *(Neurologic Clinics of North America 14, pp. 594–596, 1996)*

28. B. Clinical manifestations suggest narcolepsy or cataplexy. It is important to explore whether the patient has a family history of epilepsy and if she ever had seizures. EEG is required; the presence of epileptic discharges would suggest epilepsy, but a normal EEG does not exclude epilepsy. Monitor blood pressure in standing and recumbent positions, as this episode could represent postural hypotension or vasovagal syncope. *(Neurologic Clinics of North America 14, p. 548, 1996)*

29. D. If we assume that attacks are narcolepsy-cataplexy, stimulant and tricycle antidepressants should be initiated. Ritalin is usually utilized, but Dexedrine may also be used. Imipramine is most effective for cataplexy. Diagnosis of narcolepsy can be confirmed by multiple sleep latency study after a full-night polysomnogram has been done to exclude other sleep disorders. In narcolepsy, patients enter REM sleep stage early after falling asleep. *(Ref. 2, pp. 742–745)*

30. A. Hypnogogic hallucinations and sleep paralysis are part of the narcolepsy syndrome. Obtain serum potassium to exclude hypokalemic periodic paralysis as the cause of sudden loss of muscle tone. *(Ref. 2, p. 742)*

31. D. In REM behavior disorder, there is motor activity which may be violent in nature; this occurs during REM sleep. There is incomplete maintenance of REM atonia which may affect the arms, legs, and face. This may permit dream enactment, resulting in injury to the patient or his or her bed partner. This condition may be differentiated from sleep-walking because REM behavior disorder occurs later in the night (when REM sleep is more frequent) and may be associated with vivid dream recall. Fugue states do not usually occur during sleep. Obstructive sleep apnea is associated with multiple nocturnal awakenings but *not* violent behavior. *(Ref. 2, p. 748)*

32. B. A polysomnogram is the diagnostic study to show if attacks occur during REM sleep and if EMG shows lack of atonia. If seizures are suspected, EEG would be helpful. *(Ref. 2, p. 748)*

33. D. All benzodiazepines and carbamazepine have been effective in controlling REM behavior disorder. *(Ref. 2, p. 748)*

10

DEMENTIA AND NEUROBEHAVIORAL DISORDERS

Multiple Choice

Choose the most appropriate response.

1. _____ Left handedness, or family history of left handedness, may have the following effect on language function after left hemisphere stroke:

   A. No effect
   B. Makes recovery less likely
   C. Makes recovery more likely
   D. Prevents aphasia
   E. Makes right-sided weakness less likely in association with aphasia

2. _____ H.R. is a 68-year-old man who goes to the emergency room with difficulty speaking and with right-sided weakness. On examination, his speech is non-fluent, with some word-finding difficulty. He makes some paraphasic errors and has difficulty with repetition. Comprehension is relatively preserved. What type of aphasia does he have?

   A. Wernicke aphasia
   B. Transcortical motor aphasia
   C. Broca aphasia
   D. Anomic aphasia
   E. None of the above

3. _____ The following is a feature of Gerstmann syndrome:

   A. Aphasia
   B. Agraphia
   C. Apraxia
   D. Alexia
   E. Anosagnosia of Babinski

4. _____ The following vascular lesion can cause cognitive impairment:

   A. Left capsular lacunar infarct
   B. Left middle cerebral artery branch occlusion
   C. Right posterior parietal hemorrhage
   D. Unruptured carotid berry aneurysm
   E. None of the above

5. _____ The following agents slow the pathological progression of Alzheimer's disease:

   A. Trental
   B. Hydergine
   C. Deprenyl
   D. Cognex
   E. None of the above

6. _____ The following is true of cobalamin deficiency:

   A. Patients may initially present with acral numbness and paresthesias
   B. Syncope and fatigue may be initial symptoms
   C. Myelopathy and neuropathy may both be seen on clinical exam
   D. Psychoses may develop
   E. All of the above

7. _____ In patients with Alzheimer's disease:

   A. EEG shows paroxysmal lateralizing epileptiform discharges (PLEDS)
   B. CSF shows pleocytosis
   C. MRI shows left temporal atrophy
   D. CT shows meningeal enhancement
   E. SPECT shows bilateral decreased temporal-parietal perfusion

8. _____ This clinical feature is unique to all perisylvian aphasias:

   A. Impaired repetition
   B. Anomia
   C. Agraphia
   D. Nonfluent paraphasic speech
   E. Impaired comprehension

9. _____ The most appropriate definition of apraxia is:

   A. Inability to recognize objects
   B. Impaired comprehension
   C. Impaired speech output
   D. Inability to perform learned task with normal strength, coordination, and comprehension
   E. Impaired articulation

10. _____ A 70-year-old woman develops increasing forgetfulness and has word-finding difficulty. This apolipoprotein E pattern is most suggestive of Alzheimer's disease as the cause of the neurological disturbances:

    A. E2/E2
    B. E2/E3
    C. E3/E3
    D. E3/E4
    E. E4/E4

11. _____ Characteristics of global aphasia include:

    A. Nonfluent speech
    B. Impaired repetition
    C. Impaired comprehension
    D. Anomia
    E. All of the above

12. _____ Characteristics of transcortical motor aphasia include:

    A. Nonfluent speech, intact repetition and comprehension, anomia
    B. Fluent anomic speech with normal comprehension
    C. Nonfluent anomic speech with impaired repetition
    D. Alexia with agraphia
    E. Dysarthric anomic speech with poor repetition

13. _____ Clinical features of normal-pressure hydrocephalus (NPH) include:

    A. Dementia
    B. Gait apraxia
    C. Incontinence
    D. Memory impairment
    E. All of the above

14. _____ Clinical features of progressive supranuclear palsy (PSP) include:

    A. Impaired horizontal eye movements
    B. 3-cps resting tremor
    C. Dysmetria
    D. Truncal rigidity, impaired vertical eye movements, cognitive-behavioral disorders
    E. Diplopia

15. _____ An effective medication to treat visual hallucinations in Parkinson's patients who require Sinemet is:

    A. Cogentin
    B. Clozapine
    C. Haldol
    D. Thorazine
    E. Mellaril

16. _____ Subcortical dementia is seen in this disorder:

    A. Huntington's disease
    B. Wilson's disease
    C. Parkinson's disease
    D. Progressive supranuclear palsy
    E. All of the above

17. _____ The following statements are true of Binswanger's disease:

    A. Acute strokes occur throughout natural history
    B. Seizures and dementia occur
    C. CT/MRI show periventricular white-matter lesions
    D. Pathology shows hyalinized arteries within the white matter
    E. All of the above

18. _____ These drugs may interfere with motor recovery in stroke patients:

    A. Clonidine
    B. Valproic acid
    C. Haloperidol
    D. Phenytoin
    E. All of the above

19. _____ Neuropathological lesions may be found in this region in patients with obsessive-compulsive behavior (OCB):

    A. Frontal lobe
    B. Temporal lobe
    C. Cerebellum
    D. Parietal lobe
    E. None of the above

20. _____ The following drugs—alone or in combination—may cause "serotonin syndrome":

    A. Meperidine
    B. Phenelzine
    C. L-tryptophan
    D. Sumatriptan
    E. All of the above

21. _____ Diagnostic criteria for dementia include:

    A. Loss of intellectual capability of such magnitude as to interfere with activities of daily living
    B. Impaired memory, abstraction, problem solving, constructional ability, and personality change
    C. No evidence of delirium until later stages of illness
    D. All of the above
    E. None of the above

22. _____ In patients with Alzheimer's disease, this pathological finding may be present:

A. Negri bodies
B. Cowdry inclusion bodies
C. Lewy bodies
D. None of the above
E. All of the above

23. _____ Cerebral blood flow and metabolism are decreased in Alzheimer's disease due to the following factor:

A. Ischemia
B. Reduced neuronal activity
C. Demyelination
D. Edema
E. Gliosis

24. _____ In *normal* elderly patients, examination may show the following abnormality:

A. Diminished proprioception in legs
B. Decreased vibration sensation at toes
C. Parkinsonian features
D. Fasciculations, wasting and weakness in the shoulders
E. Anosagnosia

25. _____ Symptoms of neuroleptic malignant syndrome include:

A. Motor rigidity
B. Hyperthermia
C. Rhabdomyolysis
D. Delirium
E. All of the above

26. _____ Treatment of neuroleptic malignant syndrome includes:

A. Bromocriptine
B. Physostigmine
C. Acetylsalicylic acid
D. Acetaminophen
E. Reserpine

27. _____ Triazolam (Halcion) may produce this syndrome:

A. Status epilepticus
B. Transient ischemic attack
C. Transient global amnesia (TGA)
D. Broca aphasia
E. Amaurosis

28. _____ Drug intoxication should not be suspected in a comatose patient with the following neurological features:

A. Focal neurological signs
B. Asymmetrical, unequal pupils
C. Dysconjugate eye movements
D. Unilateral Babinski sign
E. All of the above

29. _____ These eye movements may be seen in drug intoxication:

A. Ophthalmoplegia
B. Forced downward ocular deviation opsoclonus
C. Nystagmus
D. Opsoclonus
E. None of the above

Matching

Match the clinical feature with the dementia etiology.

A. Myoclonus
B. Gait apraxia
C. Argyll-Robertson pupils
D. Pseudobulbar palsy
E. Chorea

30. _____ Normal-pressure hydrocephalus (NPH)

31. _____ Huntington's disease (HD)

32. _____ Neurosyphilis (NS)

33. _____ Jakob-Creutzfeldt disease (J-C)

34. _____ Multiinfarct dementia (MID)

Match the CT finding with the dementia type.

A. Enlarged ventricles and subarachnoid spaces
B. Enlarged ventricles and poorly visualized cortical and basal cisternal spaces
C. Semilunar hypodense extracerebral lesions
D. "Squared out" caudate nuclei
E. Hypodensities in basal ganglia

35. _____ Wilson's disease

36. _____ Huntington's disease (HD)

37. _____ Alzheimer's disease (NPH)

38. _____ Normal-pressure hydrocephalus

39. _____ Bilateral subdural hematomas

Multiple Choice

Choose the most appropriate response.

A 28-year-old HIV-positive homosexual man complains of difficulty sleeping and problems with memory and thinking. He reports difficulty with concentration and cannot remember what he recently read in the newspaper. He says he is afraid he will lose his keys, forget to pay bills, or leave the oven on; however, he has *not* done any of these things. Medication includes AZT only. He has had no opportunistic infections. Neurological examination including mini-mental status shows no abnormality.

40. _____ What is the most likely diagnosis?

A. AIDS dementia
B. AZT-induced cognitive impairment
C. Neurosyphilis
D. Affective disorder
E. Cryptococcal meningitis

41. _____ Lumbar puncture is performed and there are 30 lymphocytes and a protein content of 80 mg% with no other abnormalities. What is the most likely diagnosis?

A. AIDS-dementia complex
B. Toxoplasmosis
C. Neurosyphilis
D. Cryptococcal meningitis
E. Not enough information to establish diagnosis

42. _____ What should the next neurodiagnostic test be?

A. CT
B. MRI
C. Neuropsychological testing
D. EEG
E. Further CSF studies

43. _____ Six months later the patient reported that he experienced numbness in both hands but that no numbness was present in his feet. Examination showed reduced pinprick in his thumb and index fingers and positive Tinel sign. What is the most likely diagnosis?

A. AZT neuropathy
B. AIDS neuropathy
C. Cervical radiculopathy
D. Carpal tunnel syndrome
E. All of the above

A 65-year-old woman with no cardiovascular or cerebrovascular history complains of memory impairment. She forgets to pay her bills and gets lost driving home. She becomes anxious and reports that people are walking through her house when no one else can confirm this suspicion. Examination shows mild memory impairment, concreteness of thought, word-finding difficulty, and paranoid ideation. The remainder of the exam is normal.

44. _____ Based on the history as given, what is the most likely diagnosis?

A. Affective disorder
B. Dementia of Alzheimer's type
C. Huntington's disease
D. Diffuse Lewy body disease
E. Multiinfarct dementia

45. _____ What should be the initial diagnostic test?

A. EEG
B. LP
C. CT
D. MRI
E. None of the above

46. _____ She is treated with Cognex and Haldol. Following this, she reports difficulty with walking and right-arm resting tremor. What is the most likely diagnosis?

A. Cerebral infarct
B. Drug-induced Parkinsonism
C. Huntington's disease
D. Cognex-induced dyskinesia
E. None of the above

47. _____ While she receives Cognex and Haldol, which laboratory studies need to be monitored serially?

A. Liver function
B. CPK
C. Renal function
D. CBC
E. Platelets

48. _____ One week after initiating Cognex and Haldol, she becomes febrile, stiff, and disoriented. What is the most likely diagnosis?

A. Malignant neuroleptic syndrome (MNS)
B. Pneumonia
C. Cognex drug effect
D. Meningitis
E. None of the above

49. _____ Which laboratory study is most likely to be abnormal in this condition (see Question 48)?

A. CPK
B. Liver function
C. EEG
D. LP
E. CBC

RESPONSES AND EXPLANATIONS

1. **C.** Right-handed people are almost always left-hemispheric dominant. With left-handed people, the situation is more complex. Approximately 70% of left-handed people are *still* left-hemispheric dominant; whereas the others are right-hemispheric or mixed dominant. If the patient is mixed dominant, language is less severely affected following left-hemispheric stroke. To determine hemispheric dominance, inject amobarbital into each carotid artery to determine the effect on language (Wada test). When amobarbital is injected into the language-dominant hemisphere, the patient becomes aphasic. This test is important to perform in patients who will undergo temporal lobectomy for medically intractable seizures to assess hemispheric dominance for language. *(Ref. 1, pp. 854–856; Ref. 2, p. 421)*

2. **D.** Difficulty with spontaneous speech and impaired repetition with intact comprehension define Broca aphasia. In transcortical motor and anomic aphasia, repetition remains intact. *(Ref. 1, pp. 8–11; Ref. 2, pp. 421–423)*

3. **B.** Gerstmann syndrome is defined by
   a. Right–left confusion
   b. Finger agnosia
   c. Agraphia
   d. Acalculia
   (Ref. 2, p. 426)

4. **E.** Vascular cognitive impairment (dementia) may be due to
   a. Multiple vascular lesions, e.g., infarcts or hemorrhage
   b. A single large vascular lesion
   c. Strategically placed vascular lesions, e.g., thalamic
   None of the listed lesions fits these criteria. Vascular dementia occurs in patients with stroke risk factors. Patients should experience abrupt, discrete episodes of neurological worsening. Neurological examination should show bilateral hemisphere and/or brainstem findings. Vascular dementia diagnosis is not established only by CT/MRI findings of multiple vascular-appearing ischemic lesions. *(Lancet 2, p. 207, 1976; Ref. 2. pp. 414–415)*

5. **E.** Tacrine (Cognex) may improve cognitive function *symptomatically,* but it does not halt pathological progression. Hydergine has never been shown to be effective in reversing or improving symptoms of dementia. Trental is a vasodilating and hemorheological agent but has not been shown to be effective in vascular dementia. Deprenyl is believed to be effective in PD, but there is no evidence of effectiveness in Alzheimer's disease. *(Mayo Clinic Proceedings 70, p. 1116, 1995)*

6. **E.** In subacute combined system degeneration (B_{12} deficiency), there may be peripheral nerve and spinal cord lesions. There may also be brain involvement that causes "megaloblastic madness" or dementia. Defective DNA synthesis in rapidly dividing bone marrow cells may cause fatigue and syncope. Most patients have *low* B_{12} blood levels, but if normal, check for metabolites which may be present with B_{12} deficiency, e.g., methylmalonic acid. Treat with intramuscularly administered B_{12}. *(Ref. 2, pp. 691–692)*

7. **E.** In AD, SPECT shows reduced metabolism and perfusion in the temporal and parietal regions. MRI shows *symmetrical* atrophy in AD. *(Mayo Clinic Proceedings 70, p. 1095, 1994; Ref. 1, pp. 677–685)*

8. **A.** In all perisylvian aphasias (global, conduction, Wernicke, Broca), repetition is impaired; whereas in transcortical aphasia (sensory, motor), repetition is *normal.* *(Ref. 2, pp. 421–423)*

9. **D.** Apraxia for gait or dressing involves failure to perform learned motor tasks due to a defect in executive motor planning. *(Ref. 1, pp. 8–11; Ref. 2, pp. 423–427)*

10. **E.** A double dose of E-4 is the most likely pattern to be associated with cognitive impairment due to AD; however, if a patient has this pattern but is neurologically normal, it does not necessarily mean that dementia will develop. *(Mayo Clinic Proceedings 70, p. 1093, 1995; Annals of Neurology 34, p 752, 1993; Ref. 1, pp. 677–685)*

11. **E.** Global aphasia combines the features of Wernicke and Broca aphasia. Patients have impaired comprehension with nonfluent, nonspontaneous speech. *(Ref. 1, pp. 8–11; Ref. 2, pp. 421–422)*

12. **A.** Transcortical motor aphasia has features of Broca aphasia but with intact repetition. It develops due to ischemia in the border zone of the middle and anterior cerebral arteries. Transcortical sensory aphasia has features of Wernicke aphasia with normal repetition. This condition is due to ischemia in the border zone between the middle and posterior cerebral arteries. *(Ref. 1, pp. 8–11; Ref. 2, p. 422)*

13. **E.** All are features of NPH and can be reversed by a diversionary shunt procedure. CT/MRI shows enlarged ventricles with poor visualization of cortical sulcal spaces. Neurological features also improve following LP with removal of large quantities of CSF. *(Journal of Neurology, Neurosurgery and Psychiatry 57, p. 1021, 1991; Ref. 2, pp. 417–418)*

14. **D.** Clinical features of PSP include:
   a. Truncal and extremity rigidity
   b. Tremor not present
   c. Bradykinesia
   d. Pseudobulbar palsy
   e. Impaired vertical gaze
   f. Subcortical dementia
   (Neurology 38, p. 1031, 1988)

15. **B.** Clozapine is the neuroleptic of choice to treat hallucinations due to Sinemet in PD patients. It does not worsen or exacerbate extrapyramidal features. Mellaril is the second choice because it has the least tendency to exacerbate extrapyramidal features. It is important to be aware that Sinemet-induced visual hallucinations are not frightening or threatening to the patient, and some patients require no treatment other than reassurance. *(Ref. 1, p. 728)*

16. **E.** In cortical dementia, motor, speech, and reflex abnormalities are lacking; these disturbances are present in subcortical dementias. All the listed conditions cause subcortical dementia. *(Annals of Neurology 19, p. 1, 1986)*

17. **E.** In Binswanger's disease, there are thickened hyalinized arteries in the white matter and subcortical gray matter. Clinical features indicate multiinfarct dementia. MRI findings support the diagnosis, but Binswanger's disease is not a neuroradiological diagnosis in the absence of clinical findings to support the diagnosis. *(Neurology 45, p. 626, 1995)*

18. **E.** Certain commonly utilized neurological, psychiatric, and cardiovascular drugs may have a negative effect on motor recovery by virtue of antidopaminergic or GABA-enhancing effects. Adrenergic drugs such as Ritalin may enhance motor recovery. It is possible that drugs facilitating motor recovery may enhance alternative neural pathways to perform functions lost due to stroke. *(Stroke 21, p. 1636, 1990)*

19. **A.** Most models of OCB have implicated abnormalities in the frontal lobe, basal ganglia, and limbic structures. Functional neuroimaging has shown *hypermetabolic* abnormalities in the orbitofrontal, cingulate, and caudate regions. OCB may have structural correlates, and this should be looked for especially in those patients with other abnormal neurological signs. *(Ref. 5, pp. 193–194)*

20. **E.** This may include altered consciousness, autonomic instability, and enhanced motor activity (hyperreflexia, Babinski sign, fasciculations, myoclonus). There is usually no hyperthermia or rigidity, which helps to differentiate this from malignant neuroleptic syndrome. Be careful in migraine patients who may receive MAO or SSRI as migraine prophylaxis plus Imitrex for abortive treatment in acute attacks. *(American Journal of Psychiatry 148, p. 6, 1991)*

21. **D.** All are features of dementia, which is defined as loss or impairment of cognitive skills usually associated with behavioral disorders. Agitated confusion (delirium) may develop in demented patients when there is an intervening infection, toxic, or metabolic disorder. *(Ref. 2, pp. 408–412)*

22. **C.** Lewy body disease is a parkinsonian syndrome with or without dementia. This may be a "variant" of Alzheimer's disease. These inclusion bodies are seen in the cerebral cortex and brainstem. Characteristic pathological features of AD are senile amyloid plaques and neurofibrillary tangles. Biochemically, in AD there is reduction in choline acetyltransferase in the cerebral cortex and hippocampus. *(Neurology 40, p. 1, 1990)*

23. **B.** The brain *autoregulates* cerebral blood flow; therefore when brain atrophy occurs, there is reduced neuronal activity and reduced cerebral blood flow (CBF). The reduced CBF is a *secondary* process; therefore increasing CBF will *not* be effective therapy in AD. *(Ref. 2, pp. 414–415)*

24. **B.** In elderly patients, the following neurological features may occur in the absence of neurological illness:
    a. Hand muscle wasting
    b. Absent ankle reflexes
    c. Reduced pupillary light response
    d. Reduced vibration sensation in feet and ankles
    e. Presence of primitive reflexes (snout, grasp, palmomental)
    f. Stooped simian posture
    g. Reduced hearing, smell and vision
    (Ref. 1, pp. 1–7; Ref. 2, pp. 18–19, 34–35)

25. **E.** This is precipitated by dopamine-blocking medication. Autonomic instability (tachycardia, hypertension, diaphoresis) and elevated CPK also occur. *(Ref. 1, pp. 728, 733, 788; Ref. 2, pp. 519, 649)*

26. **A.** Treatment includes:
    a. Stop causal medication
    b. Adequate hydration
    c. Control of hyperthermia
    d. Bromocriptine
    e. Dantrolene
    (Archives of Internal Medicine 149, p. 1927, 1989)

27. **C.** Sedative-hypnotic medication may cause transient memory impairment, e.g., TGA. The mechanism of TGA may be electrical or vascular. This is a self-limited event which does *not* usually recur. Neurodiagnostic studies (EEG, CT, MRI, vascular imaging) are normal. *(Brain 113, p. 639, 1990; Ref. 1, pp. 872–873)*

28. **E.** Drug intoxication may cause metabolic encephalopathy, but there are never *focal* neurological signs. In certain metabolic encephalopathies which occur in patients who have had prior focal brain injury, e.g., stroke, contusion, with *prior* focal deficit, there may be *worsening* or *reappearance* of this focal deficit when metabolic disturbance occurs. This focal deficit resolves when the metabolic imbalance resolves. Be certain that the drug does not directly affect the pupils, e.g., heroin. *(Ref. 2, pp. 229–236)*

29. **C.** Many drugs (especially sedative-hypnotic medications) may cause nystagmus but not other the listed abnormal eye movements. *(Ref. 2, pp. 235–237)*

30. B
31. E
32. C
33. A
34. D

30–34. In AD, dementia is usually not accompanied by other neurological findings. If the patient has dementia *plus* other findings, consider alternative etiologies: for NPH, gait apraxia, spasticity, Babinski signs; for HD, chorea and hypotonia; for neurosyphilis, Argyll-Robertson pupils, abnormal reflexes and sensation due to tabes dorsalis, optic atrophy, stroke syndromes; for J-C disease, myoclonus and periodic EEG; for MID, signs of bilateral strokes including pseudobulbar palsy. *(Ref. 1, pp. 677–685)*

35. E
36. D
37. A
38. B
39. C

35–39. In AD, there is symmetrical enlargement of the ventricles and subarachnoid spaces. In Wilson's disease, necrotic and cystic lesions occur in the globus pallidus and putamen, causing hypodensities in the basal ganglia. In HD, there is bilateral caudate atrophy. In NPH, ventricles are enlarged with no visualization of cortical sulcal spaces, and periventricular hypodensities may be seen. With bilateral subdural hematomas, there may be isodense or hypodense extracerebral lesions with no visualization of cisternal or sulcal spaces, and ventricles appear small and compressed. *(Mayo Clinic Proceedings 70, p. 1093, 1995; Ref. 1, pp. 677–685; Ref. 2, pp. 408–428)*

40. A. Neurological manifestations of HIV infection occur when the patient has AIDS-defining opportunistic infections. This patient has none and is seropositive and otherwise asymptomatic. It is impossible to establish a diagnosis of dementia with an entirely normal mental state. The patient appears to have depression (affective disorder) with cognitive inefficiency of depressive illness. *(Ref. 2, pp. 476–479)*

41. E. In early stages of HIV infection, 33% of neurologically *asymptomatic* patients will have pleocytosis and elevated protein. However, more studies need to be done on CSF to exclude other conditions such as neurosyphilis, fungal tuberculous, or lymphomatous meningitis. *(Ref. 2, pp. 476–479)*

42. E. More complete CSF studies need to be done, including but not limited to:
   a. Acid fast stain
   b. Cryptococcal antigen
   c. India ink preparation
   d. p24 antigen
   e. Immunoglobulins
   f. Cytology for neoplastic cells
   g. Cultures
   (Ref. 2, pp. 476–479, 537–550)

43. D. Sensory findings in the hands without involvement of the feet is *not* consistent with polyneuropathy. Consider carpal tunnel or cervical radiculopathy (less common). This would be unrelated to HIV infection. Remember that patients with HIV infection may develop neurological abnormalities *not* related to the primary HIV infection. *(Ref. 2, pp. 476–479)*

44. B. Cognitive impairment with behavioral disorder suggests AD, but the rapid course with psychoses should raise suspicion of HD even though no chorea is described but may develop later. Examination must look carefully for subtle signs of chorea, such as tics, jitteriness, or fidgetiness. *(Ref. 1, pp. 695–699; Ref. 2, pp. 637–638)*

45. C. Noncontrast CT should be the initial study. In 80% of patients, dementia due to AD shows characteristic brain atrophy as manifested by enlarged ventricles and subarachnoid spaces. In 10% of AD patients, CT is normal. In 10% of *normals*, CT shows evidence of "cerebral atrophy." *(Ref. 1, pp. 677–685)*

46. B. Drug-induced PD has developed. Since there is no chorea, the dyskinesia does not suggest HD. *(Ref. 2, pp. 646–647)*

47. A. Tacrine (Cognex) may cause hepatic toxicity, and the liver function tests need to be carefully monitored. *(Mayo Clinic Proceedings 70, p. 1116, 1995)*

48. A. MNS develops in patients receiving dopamine-blocking agent; however, LP with CSF examination should be done to exclude meningitis. In meningitis, neck flexion is impaired; whereas in MNS, the entire body has increased tone. *(Archives of Internal Medicine 149, p. 1927, 1989)*

49. A. In MNS, muscle breakdown may cause marked elevation of CPK. More severe muscle breakdown may lead to myoglobinuria. *(Archives of Internal Medicine 49, p. 1927, 1989)*

11

CENTRAL NERVOUS SYSTEM NEOPLASMS

Matching

Match the clinical feature with the neoplasm.

A. Commonly extraaxial location originating from arachnoid granulations
B. Commonly contains a hemorrhagic component
C. Radiosensitive neoplasm which sometimes contains a hemorrhagic component
D. Large cystic component with a small mural nodule
E. Associated with von Recklinghausen's disease, especially when bilateral

1. _____ Acoustic neuroma

2. _____ Cerebellar astrocytoma

3. _____ Meningioma

4. _____ Metastatic melanoma

5. _____ Pituitary adenoma

Match the common presenting clinical feature with the neoplasm.

A. Parinaud syndrome
B. Bitemporal superior quadrantanopia
C. Bitemporal inferior quadrantanopia
D. Precocious puberty
E. Psychoses

6. _____ Bifrontal meningioma

7. _____ Hypothalamic hamartoma

8. _____ Craniopharyngioma

9. _____ Pituitary adenoma

10. _____ Pinealoma

Match the clinical feature with the neoplasm.

A. Gait ataxia
B. Unilateral visual loss and afferent pupillary defect
C. Facial pain
D. Acromegaly
E. Seizures
F. Nonlocalized intracranial hypertension

11. _____ Nasopharyngioma

12. _____ Colloid cyst of the third ventricle

13. _____ Optic glioma

14. _____ Pituitary adenoma

15. _____ Meningioma

16. _____ Medulloblastoma

Multiple Choice

Choose the most appropriate response.

17. _____ Most common neoplasm to cause amenorrhea-galactorrhea, but shows no visual disturbance.

   A. Parasellar meningioma
   B. Craniopharyngioma
   C. Pituitary microadenoma
   D. Chordoma
   E. Parasellar aneurysm

18. _____ Commonly calcified intracranial neoplasm.

   A. Low-grade glioma
   B. Oligodendroglioma
   C. Pituitary adenoma
   D. Acoustic neuroma
   E. Medulloblastoma

19. _____ The following is true of central nervous system lymphomas:

A. May arise in the absence of systemic lymphoma
B. May involve brain parenchyma, vitreous or retina of the eye
C. May occur in nonimmunosuppressed patients
D. May cause lymphomatous meningitis
E. All of the above

20. _____ In a patient with lung carcinoma who develops bilateral symmetrical cerebellar syndrome and has normal CT and MRI, this study may be helpful:

A. EMG/NCV
B. CSF
C. Anti-Purkinje cell antibody titer
D. Myelogram
E. MRI with contrast

21. _____ The most common cerebellar tumor in adults is:

A. Multiple sclerosis
B. Hemangioblastoma
C. Meningioma
D. Glioblastoma
E. Craniopharyngioma

22. _____ The type of cerebral edema caused by glioblastoma multiforme is:

A. Cytotoxic
B. Vasogenic
C. Interstitial
D. Hydrocephalic
E. All of the above

Answer based on the clinical history.

H.R. has breast cancer and is treated with simple mastectomy and irradiation. She is considered "cured." Five years later, she develops headache which awakens her from sleep, lasts 40 min, and is associated with vomiting and visual obscurations. It occurs one to three times per day. She had migraine as adolescent. Her neurological examination is normal. She has no systemic signs of cancer recurrence.

23. _____ The headache is most characteristic of:

A. Migraine
B. Cluster
C. Intracranial hypertension
D. Systemic arterial hypertension
E. Tension

24. _____ Diagnostic possibilities include:

A. Single brain metastasis
B. Multiple brain metastases
C. Carcinomatous meningitis
D. Meningioma
E. All of the above

25. _____ Management should be:

A. Treat prophylactically for migraine
B. Refer to psychiatrist
C. LP
D. Noncontrast MRI
E. Postcontrast CT

A 28-year-old schizophrenic woman develops discharge from her breasts and her menses become irregular. Her dose of Haldol is 10 mg po bid. Prolactin level is 850 (markedly elevated). Following reduction in Haldol level, galactorrhea persists and she reports visual blurring. Exam shows superior bitemporal quadrantanopia.

26. _____ The most likely diagnosis is:

A. Drug-induced galactorrhea
B. Pituitary microadenoma
C. Pituitary macroadenoma
D. Craniopharyngioma
E. Parasellar meningioma

27. _____ The neural structure which is being compressed, causing visual dysfunction in this patient, is the:

A. Optic nerve
B. Cavernous sinus
C. Optic chiasm
D. Optic radiation
E. Occipital cortex

28. _____ The most sensitive study to diagnose the cause of the visual and endocrine symptoms in this patient is:

A. MRI
B. CT
C. Skull radiogram
D. Angiogram
E. Visual field examination

29. _____ Treatment should include:

A. Discontinue Haldol
B. Bromocriptine
C. Bifrontal craniotomy
D. Transphenoidal microsurgical tumor resection
E. Irradiation therapy

30. _____ If the pituitary mass extended laterally, it would compress this structure:

    A. Cavernous sinus
    B. Frontal lobe
    C. Optic nerve
    D. Hypothalamus
    E. Brainstem

T.P. is a 46-year-old surgeon who experiences a 2-min episode of confusion during which he is observed to make bizarre lip-smacking movements. He has a bad taste in his mouth prior to the episode. Following this episode, neurological exam is normal.

31. _____ The most likely explanation for this episode is:

    A. Transient global amnesia
    B. Transient ischemic attack
    C. Petit mal seizure
    D. Partial complex seizure
    E. Migraine equivalent

32. _____ What would be most useful diagnostic test to clarify the mechanism of the described episode?

    A. EEG
    B. LP
    C. Angiogram
    D. CT
    E. MRI

33. _____ If EEG shows left temporal spike and slow wave pattern, while CT and MRI are normal, initial treatment should be:

    A. Tegretol
    B. Phenobarbital
    C. Coumadin
    D. Aspirin
    E. Ticlid

34. _____ Six months later, the patient experiences a grand mal seizure. Exam shows word-finding difficulty and right pronator drift. What should be the next management decision?

    A. EEG
    B. LP
    C. Angiogram
    D. Increase medication dose
    E. MRI

35. _____ What is the most common underlying neuropathological condition that causes this clinical disorder?

    A. Glioblastoma
    B. Meningioma
    C. Aneurysm
    D. Herpes simplex encephalitis
    E. Vascular malformation

RESPONSES AND EXPLANATIONS

1. **E.** Acoustic neuroma occurs as part of von Recklinghausen syndrome (neurofibromatosis), especially if the neuromas are bilateral. Neuroma begins in the vestibular portion of the eighth nerve within the internal auditory canal. It may enlarge to extend into the cerebellopontine angle. *(Ref. 1, pp. 326–328; Ref. 2, pp. 133–134)*

2. **D.** Cerebellar astrocytomas are common childhood neoplasms. They are frequently cystic and contain small mural solid nodules. These usually can be treated surgically and do not require irradiation. *(Ref. 1, p 339; Ref. 4, pp. 190–191)*

3. **A.** Meningiomas originate from arachnoid granulations. The most common sites of origin are the cerebral hemispheric dural surface. They are calcified, sharply marginated, extraaxial neoplasms, located outside the brain parenchyma. These are benign tumors which can be surgically excised because of their location; however, some may recur or undergo malignant transformation. *(Ref. 1, pp. 332–340; Ref. 2, pp. 442–448)*

4. **B.** Brain neoplasms are not commonly hemorrhagic. Primary brain neoplasms which sometimes show hemorrhage include glioblastoma multiforme and pituitary adenoma. Secondary (metastatic) neoplasms which hemorrhage include lung, melanoma, choriocarcinoma, and hypernephroma. *(Ref. 1, p. 911)*

5. **C.** Pituitary adenoma are benign juxtasellar neoplasms which are frequently highly radiosensitive. They may contain hemorrhagic or cystic components, and these are less likely to be radiosensitive. They originate from the anterior pituitary and cause endocrine and visual disturbances. *(Ref. 1, pp. 885–890; Ref. 2, pp. 444–447; Ref. 4, pp. 192–193)*

6. **E.** Bifrontal meningiomas may cause cognitive and behavioral disturbances including psychoses that simulate schizophrenia. Other patients with bifrontal meningiomas are apathetic, with psychomotor retardation, and appear depressed. *(Ref. 1, pp. 330–333)*

7. **D.** Precocious puberty refers to early onset of androgen secretion in boys and estrogen production in girls, with premature development of sexual characteristics. Hypothalamic hamartoma may cause precocious puberty and may be part of von Recklinghausen's disease. *(Ref. 1, pp. 361, 634)*

8. **C.** Craniopharyngiomas are suprasellar neoplasms that compress the upper chiasmal fibers which represent *inferior* bitemporal visual fields. These tumors occur in childhood, cause hypopituitarism, and show suprasellar calcification on skull radiogram or CT. *(Ref. 1, pp. 375–377; Ref. 2, pp. 436–437)*

9. **B.** Pituitary adenomas are intrasellar tumors which may extend to the suprasellar region. They initially compress the undersurface of the optic chiasm, causing superior bitemporal visual field defect. Some adenomas compress the normal pituitary, causing hypopituitarism; whereas others contain cells which secrete pituitary hormones, causing hyperpituitary states, e.g., prolactin-secreting tumor (galactorrhea-amenorrhea), growth hormone-secreting tumor (acromegaly), adrenocorticotropin-secreting tumor (Cushing syndrome). *(Ref. 1, pp. 367–372)*

10. **A.** Pinealoma may compress the tegmentum of the midbrain, causing inability to gaze upward. The pupils are dilated and react to accommodation but not to light (Parinaud syndrome). Tumor compression of the posterior third ventricle causes obstructive hydrocephalus. *(Ref. 1, pp. 359–367)*

11. **C.** This tumor arises in the nasopharynx adjacent to the eustachian tube in the fossa of Rosenmueller at the skull base. Common clinical symptoms include facial pain and numbness due to trigeminal nerve involvement or horizontal diplopia due to abducens nerve involvement. Diagnosis is established by examination and biopsy of the nasopharynx mass. Unexplained isolated abducens nerve paresis in an adult patient should raise clinical suspicion of nasopharyngioma. *(Ref. 1, p. 322; Ref. 5, p. 379)*

12. **F.** Colloid cysts are located in the anterior portion of the third ventricle. Symptoms include severe headache which may be modified by positional change. Initial signs may be papilledema without other localizing neurological signs. This pattern is characteristic of midline tumors which cause ventricular obstruction, e.g., hydrocephalus and intracranial hypertension. *(Ref. 1, pp. 381–382; Ref. 2, p. 450)*

13. **B.** Optic glioma occurs in childhood. It causes visual loss progressing to blindness. It presents as an orbital mass which causes enlargement of the optic foramina. It may occur in patients with von Recklinghausen's disease. *(Ref. 1, p. 632; Ref. 5, p. 121, 378)*

14. **D.** Pituitary adenomas originate from adenohypophysis. Acidophilic cells may produce growth hormone (acromegaly) or prolactin (amenorrhea-galactorrhea). *(Ref. 1, pp. 885–890; Ref. 4, pp. 192–193)*

15. **E.** If meningioma originates from the dura overlying the cerebral hemispheres, seizures may be the initial symptoms. The seizures are *focal* in type. *(Ref. 2, p. 442)*

16. **A.** Medulloblastomas originate from the roof of the fourth ventricle and may then invade the cerebellar vermis. This is a childhood tumor. It grows into the fourth ventricle and infiltrates the vermis and brainstem. *(Ref. 1, p. 348; Ref. 2, p. 434)*

17. **C.** Pituitary *micro*adenoma may secrete prolactin, causing galactorrhea and amenorrhea (due to the antiestrogenic effect of prolactin). If the tumor is less than 10 mm, it remains confined to the intrasellar region and causes no visual symptoms. Other parasellar lesions may be expected to cause visual disturbances. *(Ref. 1, pp. 367–374, 885–890)*

18. **B.** Oligodendrogliomas most commonly occur in the frontal and temporal regions. These are *slow*-growing neoplasms and therefore frequently show evidence of calcification. Low-grade gliomas may also calcify but are more likely to be cystic. Craniopharyngiomas and meningiomas are neoplasms which also commonly calcify. *(Ref. 1, pp. 345–346)*

19. **E.** These originate from B-cell lymphocytes. Lymphomas may originate from periventricular, cerebellum, brainstem, or cerebral hemispheric white matter. Vitreous and retinal involvement may occur. Lymphoma may also cause meningeal spread. It is most commonly seen in immunosuppressed AIDS or transplant patients. It is highly radiosensitive and may respond to chemotherapy. *(Ref. 1, pp. 351–359)*

20. **C.** In patients with lung carcinoma who develop focal neurological deficit, brain metastases would be initially suspected, but this possibility is excluded by normal CT and MRI. Alternative diagnoses are paraneoplastic disorders including cerebellar degeneration, neuropathy, anterior horn cell disorder, and encephalomyelitis. Anti-Purkinje cell antibodies are detected in many patients with carcinomatous cerebellar degeneration. *(Ref. 1, pp. 935–945; Ref. 2, p. 452; Ref. 4, pp. 196–197)*

21. **B.** Hemangioblastomas are cystic cerebellar tumors. They may be associated with retinal angiomas or, hepatic and pancreatic cysts (von Hippel-Lindau disease). Some patients have polycythemia due to production of an erythropoietic factor by the tumor. MRI and angiogram show characteristic findings. *(Ref. 1, pp. 385–386)*

22. **B.** Vasogenic edema due to breakdown of the blood–brain barrier is most commonly seen with malignant neoplasms. This may respond to treatment with high-dose corticosteroids. *(Ref. 1, pp. 302–306; Ref. 4, pp. 198–199)*

23. **C.** Headache which awakens the patient from sleep and is associated with visual obscurations is consistent with intracranial hypertension. The fluctuations in intracranial pressure cause the headache to last for 30–60 minutes and recur multiple times. Despite normal neurological examination, diagnostic evaluation should be initiated. *(Ref. 2, pp. 108–109)*

24. **E.** Brain and meningeal metastases could cause these clinical symptoms. There is increased incidence of meningioma in patients with breast carcinoma. *(Ref. 1, pp. 395–405; Ref. 4, pp. 196–199)*

25. **E or C.** In patients with suspected intracranial neoplasm, *postcontrast* CT or MRI should be performed. If carcinomatous meningitis is suspected, LP with CSF examination including cytology should be performed. *(Ref. 1, pp. 395–405; Ref. 5, pp. 342–347)*

26. **C.** Neuroleptic medication may cause mild elevation of serum prolactin and galactorrhea. It would be expected that this value would normalize with discontinuation of Haldol. The finding of visual field defect which is characteristic of optic chiasmal compression makes diagnosis of pituitary macroadenoma most likely. Other parasellar lesions may elevate prolactin level mildly but usually not to the level seen in this patient. *(Ref. 1, pp. 885–890)*

27. **C.** The visual symptoms are due to compression of the undersurface of the optic chiasm. *(Ref. 1, pp. 368–369; Ref. 2, pp. 202–203)*

28. **A.** To visualize intra- and suprasellar extension of pituitary adenoma, *coronal* MRI sections are most useful. *(Ref. 2, pp. 70–72)*

29. **D.** In pituitary *micro*adenomas which secrete prolactin but have *no* visual signs, bromocriptine may lower the prolactin level. For pituitary *macro*adenomas that cause chiasmal compression, surgical decompression of the optic chiasm and tumor removal may be achieved with transsphenoidal microsurgical resection; however, if the tumor has *extensive* suprasellar extension, bifrontal craniotomy may be needed. Following optic chiasmal decompression, irradiation therapy should be performed, as pituitary adenomas are highly radiosensitive. *(Ref. 1, pp. 372–374)*

30. **A.** If the tumor extends laterally into the cavernous sinus, there may be symptoms due to involvement of the oculomotor, trochlear, abducens, and ophthalmic branches of the trigeminal nerve. The carotid artery is also located within the cavernous sinus, and compression by the tumor may cause carotid occlusion. *(Ref. 1, pp. 368–369)*

31. **D.** The episode of altered consciousness with automatisms is consistent with a partial complex seizure. The bad taste represents the aura. This seizure suggests the presence of a temporal lobe lesion, and tumor (most commonly primary or metastatic neoplasm) would be the most likely possibility in a patient of this age. *(Ref. 2, pp. 333–335)*

32. **A.** EEG should be performed to localize the presence of the abnormal electrical discharges, which most probably originate from the temporal lobe. *(Ref. 2, pp. 333–335)*

33. **A.** The clinical and EEG findings are consistent with a partial complex seizure originating from the left temporal lobe. Tegretol should be utilized to control seizures. It is expected that there is an underlying structural lesion despite negative

MRI/CT at the time of the initial clinical presentation. Because of high clinical suspicion of an underlying mass, reassessment would be warranted in several months or if the seizure pattern or neurological examination findings change. *(Ref. 2, pp. 333–335)*

34. **E.** As seizures change in *pattern* and examination shows Broca aphasia and right hemiparesis, *reassessment* with repeat MRI is warranted. *(Ref. 4, pp. 158–161)*

35. **A.** In a middle-aged patient who has no evidence of systemic illness, primary brain neoplasm is the most likely cause of this clinical disorder. Aneurysm and vascular malformation are unlikely to cause progressive deterioration, as they would cause intracerebral or subarachnoid hemorrhage. When meningioma becomes symptomatic, CT or MRI always shows the lesion; however, glioblastoma may not always be detected on initial CT/MRI. *(Ref. 4, pp. 186–187)*

12

CENTRAL NERVOUS SYSTEM INFECTIONS (INCLUDING AIDS)

True or False

1. _____ Toxoplasmosis is the most common cause of a brain abscess in AIDS patients. It is also a common etiology for CNS infection in transplant patients who receive immunosuppressive medication.

2. _____ Dementia and motor dysfunction may be caused by HIV even if the patient has no evidence of opportunistic infection.

3. _____ Botulism may cause progressive weakness with ocular, bulbar, and extremity involvement.

4. _____ In children, *Hemophilus influenzae* is the most common cause of viral meningitis.

5. _____ *Streptococcus pneumoniae* is the most common cause of chronic meningitis in adults.

6. _____ In immunocompromised patients, *Listeria monocytogenes* is a common cause of bacterial meningitis.

7. _____ In elderly and pediatric patients with fever who are suspected of having meningitis, Brudzinski and Kernig signs may be absent; therefore LP should still be performed in these patients even if nuchal rigidity is absent.

8. _____ In uncomplicated meningitis, papilledema is not an uncommon finding.

9. _____ A positive particle agglutination test is pathognomonic of partially treated bacterial meningitis, as this test permits identification of bacterial CSF antigens.

10. _____ In patients with acute bacterial meningitis, treatment with intravenous antibiotics for 1 week followed by oral high-dose antibiotics for 1 additional week constitutes adequate therapy.

11. _____ The occurrence of recurrent bacterial meningitis suggests the possibility of abnormal communication with subarachnoid spaces, e.g., skull fracture with otorrhea, a parameningeal source of infection, or immunosuppressed status in the patient.

12. _____ Tuberculous meningitis is an acute fulminant disorder in which seizures are a common initial presenting symptom.

Multiple Choice

Choose the most correct response.

13. _____ The most sensitive laboratory abnormality in establishing diagnosis of cryptococcal meningitis is:

   A. CSF lymphocytosis
   B. Presence of cryptococcal antigen
   C. Positive India ink preparation
   D. Positive cryptococcal culture
   E. Abnormal chest radiogram

14. _____ In patients with syphilitic meningitis the following is (are) true:

   A. Low titer of nonspecific reagin antibody is evidence of active disease
   B. Low titer of specific treponemal antibody is evidence of active disease
   C. High-titer VDRL is indicative of active disease
   D. All of the above
   E. None of the above

15. _____ Clinical patterns of neurosyphilis include:

   A. Meningovascular
   B. Basilar meningitis
   C. General paresis
   D. Tabes dorsalis
   E. All of the above

16. _____ Progressive multifocal leukoencephalopathy is due to infection with this virus:

   A. Papovavirus
   B. Toxoplasmosis

C. Kuru
D. Herpes zoster
E. Herpes simplex

17. _____ In patients with CNS involvement due to Lyme disease:

A. CSF shows lymphocyte cellular response
B. CSF contains anti-B burgdorferi antibodies
C. Patient may present with multiple sclerosis-like clinical picture
D. Patient may have Guillain-Barré syndrome
E. All of the above

18. _____ Tetanus toxin affects the CNS by this mechanism:

A. Blocking interneurons
B. Stimulating alpha motor neurons
C. Stimulating gamma neurons
D. Enhancing dopamine
E. Enhancing gamma-aminobutyric acid

19. _____ The diagnosis of this parasitic infection can be established by muscle biopsy:

A. Toxoplasmosis
B. Trichinosis
C. Cysticercosis
D. Malaria
E. Naegleria

20. _____ The most common neurological manifestation of HIV infection is:

A. Toxoplasmosis
B. Lymphoma
C. Dementia
D. Seizures and psychoses
E. Myelopathy

21. _____ In the very early stage of viral meningitis, cellular response may include:

A. Polymorphonuclear and lymphocyte
B. Lymphocyte alone
C. Basophil
D. Eosinophil
E. Macrophage

22. _____ Negri bodies are seen in the brain of patients with this viral disease:

A. Herpes simplex
B. Herpes zoster
C. Rabies
D. Enterovirus
E. Myxovirus

23. _____ Peripheral facial palsy may occur in patients with this disorder:

A. Diabetes mellitus
B. Sarcoidosis
C. Lyme disease
D. Leukemia
E. All of the above

24. _____ In patients with tuberculous meningitis:

A. Skin test is usually positive
B. Chest radiogram is usually abnormal
C. CSF shows lymphocytes
D. CSF sugar is decreased and protein is markedly elevated
E. All of the above

25. _____ Cysticercosis frequently causes this neurological disturbance:

A. Intracranial calcification and seizures
B. Myopathy
C. Neuropathy
D. Dementia
E. Psychosis

Respond based on the clinical history.

P.T. is a 30-year-old homosexual alcoholic male who is admitted to the hospital confused, delirious, and tremulous. He has fever of 39°C, pulse of 110, and appears diaphoretic. He reports tactile hallucinations. Examination shows asterixis. He has negative Kernig and Brudzinski sign.

26. _____ The initial diagnostic study should be:

A. Liver function tests including arterial blood ammonia
B. CT with contrast
C. EEG
D. LP
E. MRI

27. _____ Initial treatment should include:

A. Thiamine
B. Glucose-containing fluids
C. Low-protein diet
D. Librium
E. All of the above

28. _____ Diagnostic possibilities include:

A. Acute delirium tremens
B. Wernicke encephalopathy

C. Neurosyphilis
D. Progressive multifocal leukoencephalopathy
E. All of the above

I.T.T. has frontal sinusitis which is treated with nasal decongestants and oral antibiotics. He develops fever, headache, and confusion. Neurological examination shows altered mentation, papilledema, and positive Kernig sign.

29. _____ The initial diagnostic study should be:

A. CBC
B. ESR
C. Skull and sinus radiogram
D. LP
E. CT—brain

30. _____ After all these studies are done, the patient becomes confused and has fixed, dilated left pupil and right hemiparesis. What is the likely explanation?

A. Subdural hematoma
B. Postmeningitic stroke
C. Subarachnoid hemorrhage
D. Subdural empyema
E. Neurosyphilis

31. _____ The most likely explanation of neurological deterioration in this patient would be:

A. Subfalcine herniation
B. Tonsillar herniation
C. Transtentorial herniation
D. Brain infarction
E. Subarachnoid hemorrhage

32. _____ Treatment should be:

A. Observation
B. Oral high-dose antibiotics and surgery
C. Intravenous high-dose antibiotics and surgery
D. Surgery alone
E. Intravenous antibiotics

J.R. is a 13-year-old boy who develops fever, headache, and begins to "talk crazy." He acts bizarrely and urinates into a trash container. Examination shows Wernicke aphasia and right homonymous hemianopsia.

33. _____ CSF findings would most likely show:

A. Eosinophilic pleocytosis
B. Lymphocytic pleocytosis
C. Polymorphonuclear (PMN) pleocytosis
D. Elevated gamma-globulin content
E. None of the above

34. _____ CT might be expected to show:

A. Left temporal hypodense ring-enhancing lesion
B. Bitemporal hypodense nonenhancing lesions
C. Left temporal hemorrhage
D. Left temporal infarction
E. None of the above

35. _____ The next procedure should be:

A. Meningeal biopsy
B. Brain biopsy
C. Viral CSF culture
D. Bacterial CSF culture
E. Empirical Acyclovir therapy without biopsy

A 36-year-old intravenous heroin addict has left focal motor seizure. Exam shows left hemiparesis-hemianesthesia. He has heart murmur of aortic insufficiency and is febrile. CT shows multiple hypodense ring-enhancing lesions.

36. _____ The most likely diagnosis is:

A. Bacterial meningitis
B. Bacterial endocarditis with brain abscess
C. Drug-induced cerebral vasculitis
D. Subarachnoid hemorrhage
E. Ruptured mycotic aneurysm

37. _____ Treatment should include:

A. Surgical excision of abscesses
B. Corticosteroids
C. Intravenous antibiotics
D. Oral antibiotics
E. Anticoagulation

38. _____ Two days later, this patient complains of severe headache and becomes comatose. Diagnostic possibilities include:

A. Ruptured mycotic aneurysm
B. Ruptured berry aneurysm
C. Bacterial meningitis
D. Transtentorial herniation
E. Status epilepticus

39. _____ The initial diagnostic study should be:

A. Noncontrast CT
B. Postcontrast CT
C. EEG
D. Angiogram
E. LP

RESPONSES AND EXPLANATIONS

1. **T.** This is the most common AIDS-related mass lesion. Clinical features include seizures or progressive neurological deficit. CT/MRI show enhancing brain lesions. Antibodies to toxoplasmosis are present in 95% of patients; however, these antibodies may be present in many patients without toxoplasmosis. Also, toxoplasmosis is commonly seen in transplant patients who are receiving immunosuppressive medication. *(Annals of Internal Medicine 123, p. 594, 1995)*

2. **T.** AIDS-dementia complex is a progressive subcortical dementia (slowed thought processes, apathy, speech disturbances) with motor disturbances (gait apraxia, ataxia, paraparesis). Virus may be cultured from CSF. *(Lancet 348, p. 445, 1996)*

3. **T.** Botulism results from release of toxin which may develop in home-canned foods. This toxin blocks release of acetylcholine at neuromuscular junctions. Symptoms develop 6–48 hr after eating spoiled food. Initial weakness may involve lower cranial (bulbar) musculature and later spread to the limbs and trunk. Pupils are dilated and do not react to light due to parasympathetic blockage. The toxin is destroyed by heat (cooking). Use of trivalent antitoxin and gastrointestinal lavage should be carried out in suspected individuals. *(Ref. 1, pp. 224–225)*

4. **F.** *H. influenzae* is a common type of *bacterial* meningitis which occurs in infants and children. Subdural effusion may develop with any acute bacterial meningitis but is most common with this organism. This organism is usually ampicillin sensitive, but now third-generation cephalosporins are more reliable because ampicillin-resistant strains have developed. *(Ref. 1, pp. 110–111; Ref. 2, pp. 537–550)*

5. **F.** *S. pneumoniae* (pneumococcus) is the most common etiology of *acute* meningitis in immunocompetent adults. Treatment should be *intravenous* penicillin or ampicillin. *(Ref. 1, pp. 110–111)*

6. **T.** *Listeria* occurs in adults with chronic immunosuppressive illnesses. On Gram stain or culture, they may resemble diphtheroids. Treatment should be intravenous ampicillin rather than cephalosporins. Consider this etiology for meningitis in elderly patients and those with cancer. *(Ref. 1, p. 112)*

7. **T.** In elderly patients and some children with meningitis (usually younger than 1 year), meningeal irritation signs may not be demonstrated. In such patients, unexplained fever with or without altered mental state is an indication for LP. Be cognizant that fever alone may be present in patients with noninfectious encephalopathy; however, meningoencephalitis must be excluded by negative CSF examination if fever remains unexplained. *(Ref. 2, pp. 539–540)*

8. **F.** In meningitis, the finding of papilledema indicates the presence of a *complicating* pathological process, e.g., abscess, cerebritis, empyema, venous sinus thrombosis, hydrocephalus. Papilledema does *not* occur in uncomplicated meningitis. When it is present, lumbar puncture should be delayed due to the risk of precipitating herniation syndrome from the presence of a complicating mass lesion. Perform CT/MRI to determine the nature of the complicating pathological process before performing LP in this clinical circumstance. *(Ref. 2, p. 540)*

9. **T.** In patients with suspected bacterial meningitis who have received prior antibiotic therapy (usually administered orally or intramuscularly), Gram stain and CSF culture are usually negative because of low bacterial content. This represents partially treated bacterial meningitis, as full treatment of meningitis requires a 10- to 14-day course of *high-dose intravenous* antibiotics. With negative Gram stain and culture, it is important to distinguish bacterial meningitis from other forms of meningitis, e.g., viral, and this can be most sensitively done by demonstrating bacterial capsular antigen. *(Ref. 2, pp. 541–542)*

10. **F.** In bacterial meningitis, intravenous antibiotics must be utilized for 10–14 days. This is because the presence of the blood–brain barrier limits access of antibiotics. Prognosis for meningitis is related to how rapidly appropriate antibiotic therapy is initiated. Initiate therapy without awaiting bacteriological confirmation of *bacterial* meningitis diagnosis. If necessary, switch antibiotics based on culture and sensitivity results. *(Ref. 2, pp. 540–547)*

11. **T.** Multiple episodes of meningitis indicate a host defense defect of either immunological or anatomical type. For example, an AIDS patient with CD 4+ lymphocytic defect may develop recurrent meningitis. In addition, patients who have suffered head trauma such as basilar skull fracture may have CSF leakage due to anatomic defect, and this may lead to recurrent meningitis. In the latter patient, skull tomograms and isotope cisternogram are required to identify the location of CSF leak which is predisposing the patient to meningitis, so the leak may then be surgically repaired. *(Ref. 2, p. 547)*

12. **F.** Tuberculous meningitis is *subacute* or *chronic* and is almost never acute. In meningitis, initial symptoms are headache, fever, and meningeal irritation. When seizures or progressive neurological deficit occur, consider complicating pathological processes such as vasculitis, hydrocephalus, or a mass lesion such as tuberculoma. *(Ref. 2, pp. 549–551; Ref. 4, pp. 266–267)*

13. **B.** CSF findings are similar to those of tuberculous meningitis, with lymphocytic pleocytosis, elevated protein, and re-

duced sugar content. The presence of encapsulated organisms is seen with India ink preparation, but CSF and serum cryptococcal antigen are the most sensitive tests. Cultures of CSF, urine, sputum, and bone marrow may be positive. Skin and mucous membranes may be the primary source, but the respiratory tract is the usual portal of entry; however, chest radiogram is usually normal. One-half of cases of cryptococcal meningitis occur in immunosuppressed patients or those with systemic debilitating illness, e.g., diabetes, SLE; however, in the other half, there is no associated systemic illness identified which should predispose to cryptococcal meningitis. *(Ref. 4, pp. 268–269)*

14. **C.** Neurosyphilis results from brain, meninges, and spinal cord infection by *Treponema pallidum.* Non-treponemal antibodies react to "reagin." The VDRL test is highly specific for diagnosis of syphilis, and this titer usually falls with treatment and rises with syphilis recurrence. False-positive CSF VDRL results occur in the presence of paraproteinemias, autoimmune diseases (SLE), or contamination of CSF with blood. In the *specific* Treponemal antibody test, the antigen is made from spirochetes; however, following treatment this test remains positive and is a marker of disease *history* but not disease *activity. (Ref. 4, pp. 274–275)*

15. **E.** Clinical patterns of neurosyphilis include:
    a. Asymptomatic
    b. Meningeal
    c. Vascular
    d. Parenchymal—tabetic, general paresis, optic atrophy.
    Syphilis is a great simulator of other neurological conditions. With rising incidence of AIDS, neurosyphilis is becoming a common neurological disorder once again. *(Ref. 1, pp. 200–208)*

16. **A.** Papovavirus causes multiple demyelinated CNS lesions, usually in the subcortical white matter and especially in the parieto-occipital region. This demyelinated disorder rarely involves the spinal cord, brainstem, or optic nerve (as contrasted to multiple sclerosis). At brain biopsy or autopsy, eosinophilic intranuclear inclusion bodies are seen within enlarged, abnormal-appearing oligodendrocytes. *(Ref. 1, pp. 167–168)*

17. **E.** Lyme disease is due to the spirochete, *Borrelia burgdorferi.* Systemic manifestations include skin rash and arthritis. The disease is spread by the ixodoid tick. Neurological manifestations include radiculopathy, cranial neuropathies, encephalitis, and myelitis. CSF may show pleocytosis, oligoclonal bands, and spirochete specific antibodies. Clinical features of Lyme disease may simulate Guillain-Barré or MS. *(Ref. 4, pp. 282–283)*

18. **A.** *Clostridium tetani* produces toxin which blocks inhibitory interneurons in the spinal cord. Symptoms include generalized muscle spasms (trismus is jaw muscle spasm, risus

sardonicus is spasm of facial muscles, opisthotonus is trunk muscle spasm). If treated with antitoxin, they may neutralize toxin not yet localized within the CNS. Toxin *reversibly* binds to the CNS, as contrasted with irreversible binding which occurs with rabies virus. If respiratory and autonomic dysfunction can be minimized, the patient improves in 4–8 weeks and usually recovers. *(Ref. 4, pp. 276–277)*

19. **B or C.** *Trichinella spiralis* infection is acquired by ingesting larvae in undercooked pork. The larvae cause systemic infection (fever, myalgia, arthralgia, headache). Neurologic symptoms include headache, confusion, and seizures, with tender muscles and periorbital edema. Blood count shows leukocytosis and eosinophilia. *Muscle biopsy* may establish the diagnosis. Cysticercosis may be detected by biopsy of subcutaneous nodules or muscles. *(Ref. 1, pp. 214–215)*

20. **A.** Toxoplasmosis is the most common neurological manifestation of HIV infection. Lymphoma can be confused with toxoplasmosis by CT/MRI; therapeutic trial with antitoxoplasmosis agents (pyrimethamine and sulfadiazine) should be tried before brain biopsy. Clinical and neuroimaging improvement occur with this treatment. If improvement does not occur within 2 weeks, consider alternative diagnosis and brain biopsy. *(Lancet 348, p. 445, 1996)*

21. **A.** In almost all viral meningoencephalitis, cellular response is lymphocytic pleocytosis; however, in the very early stage, PMN cells may be seen. If there is lymphocytic pleocytosis with normal sugar and protein content, this usually means that the meningitis is of viral etiology. *(Ref. 4, pp. 270–271)*

22. **C.** Rabies is a viral illness transmitted to humans in the saliva of a rabid animal. It spreads to the CNS and causes encephalitis and myelitis. There are cytoplasmic eosinophilic inclusion bodies with central basophilic granules in the neurons (Negri bodies), usually seen in hippocampal pyramidal cells or cerebellar Purkinje cells. Paralysis is due to myelitis; coma, convulsions, and laryngeal spasm are due to encephalitis. Both passive and active immunization should be attempted; however, once the toxin binds *irreversibly* to the CNS, recovery is unlikely despite vigorous supportive care. *(Ref. 4, pp. 280–281)*

23. **A or E.** Peripheral facial paralysis involving both upper and lower face muscles may be caused by all the listed conditions. In addition, herpes zoster may cause facial paralysis; the mouth and ears should be examined for herpetic vesicles. Most cases are idiopathic (Bell's palsy), and these unusual causes should be looked for only if facial paralysis is bilateral, recurrent, or there are associated systemic or neurological symptoms. Treatment of idiopathic facial palsy includes a short course of corticosteroids. This should be avoided if the etiology is thought to be due to herpes virus, in which case Acyclovir is utilized. *(Annals of Otology, Rhinology, and Laryngology 105, p. 371, 1996)*

24. **E.** Tuberculous meningitis is subacute or chronic meningitis. It is associated with *lymphocytic* reaction with *low* sugar and frequently *markedly* increased protein content. Chest radiogram and skin test are usually but not always positive. Diagnosis may be difficult in immunosuppressed patients, e.g., those with AIDS. CSF culture to detect the organism may take 3 weeks; acid fast CSF stain should be positive. If all studies are negative but diagnosis of tuberculous meningitis is still suspected, a therapeutic trial of antituberculous medication should be tried for several months. *(Ref. 4, pp. 266–267)*

25. **A.** This is caused by encystment of larvae of pork tapeworm in human tissue. Initially, there is active inflammation; later, cyst formation, gliosis, and calcification develop. Larval forms develop in subcutaneous tissue and skeletal muscle (but myopathy does not occur); brain cysts may form in meninges, causing meningitis, mass lesions, or hydrocephalus. If cysts occur in brain, they may later calcify and seizures may develop. *(Ref. 1, pp. 214–215; Ref. 2, pp. 574–575)*

26. **A.** Because of findings that the patient is delirious and tremulous, with tactile hallucinations and autonomic disturbances with asterixis, acute delirium tremens and hepatic dysfunction would probably be the most likely diagnostic possibilities. I would perform liver function studies initially. I believe fever is part of the autonomic response of delirium tremens; however, it could represent CNS infection and LP should be considered if the patient has meningeal signs or fails to respond to treatment for DTs or hepatic encephalopathy. LP should be done *immediately* if meningeal signs are present. *(Ref. 2, pp. 410–413)*

27. **E.** This patient has an acute confusional state due to metabolic encephalopathy. Tactile hallucinations are consistent with delirium tremens. Asterixis is consistent but not specific for hepatic failure. These patients may be dehydrated, so glucose-containing fluids should be used and supplemented with thiamine (to prevent precipitating Wernicke syndrome). Low-protein diet is used for management of liver failure. Low-dose Librium should be used to control agitation due to DTs. *(Ref. 2, pp. 410–413)*

28. **A.** In acute delirium tremens, the patient is delirious, tremulous, and shows signs of autonomic overactivity. None of the signs of Wernicke syndrome are described in this patient. Neurosyphilis is diagnosed by positive blood and CSF serology. PML usually occurs in immunosuppressed patients, and visual hallucinations are more common than tactile hallucinations. Diagnosis of PML would best be established by MRI. *(Ref. 4, pp. 288–289)*

29. **E.** In patients with frontal sinusitis, subsequent development of CNS bacterial infection must be considered. If there is headache and meningeal signs only, consider meningitis and perform LP. If consciousness is altered and papilledema is present, consider structural lesions, e.g., cerebritis, abscess, empyema. In this case, LP is *contraindicated* until CT is performed and the presence and exact type of brain lesion is identified. *(Ref. 2, pp. 541–542)*

30. **D.** In the setting of probable CNS infection, consider subdural empyema. In patients with meningitis, vasculitis may occur, causing stroke, but the findings in this case are not consistent with cerebral infarction or hemorrhage. *(Ref. 2, pp. 556–557)*

31. **C.** *Transtentorial herniation*, which may be due to subdural empyema or brain abscess, best explains the neurological deterioration. The uncus of the medial temporal lobe is displaced into the tentorial notch, compressing and distorting the brainstem and resulting in *ipsilateral* oculomotor nerve paresis and *contralateral* hemiparesis. *(Ref. 1, p. 23; Ref. 2, pp. 364–365)*

32. **C.** Initiate *intravenous* antibiotics and then carry out surgical drainage of the subdural empyema. If a brain abscess is present as delineated by CT/MRI finding of ring-enhancing encapsulated mass, treatment is identical; however, if a suppurative lesion is not encapsulated, e.g., cerebritis, treat with intravenous antibiotics and utilize medical management of the cerebral edema (hyperventilation, steroids, mannitol). With cerebritis, surgery should be *avoided* until the lesion is *encapsulated*. In some cases of cerebritis, the lesion resolves with antibiotics alone. If *multiple* brain abscesses are present, avoid surgery. *(Ref. 1, pp. 117–119)*

33. **B.** The occurrence of headache and fever with abnormal behavior suggests CNS infection. Examination findings localize this dysfunction to the left temporal lobe. This suggests herpes simplex encephalitis. With viral illness, CSF usually shows lymphocytic pleocytosis. Eosinophils are seen with parasitic infection; PMN are seen with bacterial illness. Elevated gamma-globulin is seen in MS or neurosyphilis. Blood serology should be done to exclude neurosyphilis. *(Ref. 2, pp. 564–567)*

34. **B.** In herpes simplex encephalitis, CT may show uni- or bilateral temporal lobe hypodense lesions, usually with no contrast enhancement. Presence of a ring-enhancing lesion suggests abscess or neoplasm, e.g., glioma. In herpes simplex encephalitis, even though clinical features may suggest only left temporal lesion, bitemporal lesions are frequently seen by CT/MRI. *(Ref. 2, pp. 564–567)*

35. **E.** Since clinical and CT findings are very suggestive of herpes simplex encephalitis, utilize Acyclovir in dose of 10 mg/kg for 10 days. If clinical improvement does not occur, brain biopsy is warranted. *(Ref. 2, pp. 564–567)*

36. **B.** This suggests bacterial endocarditis with septic embolic stroke. This may lead to multiple brain abscesses. The hematogenously disseminated microorganisms may lodge in and weaken the arterial walls. This results in mycotic aneurysm

formation. The presence of multiple ring-enhancing lesions suggests brain abscesses. *(Ref. 1, pp. 123–124; Ref. 2, p. 715)*

37. **C.** Treatment is intravenous antibiotics. Surgery is never indicated for multiple abscesses. Heparin is not utilized for septic embolism because of the risk of precipitating brain hemorrhage due to arterial wall pathology. *(Ref. 2, p. 715)*

38. **A.** Sudden headache and coma suggest *ruptured* mycotic aneurysm. These are located at *distal* arterial sites, as contrasted with the *proximal* arterial site of a berry aneurysm. Angiography demonstrates aneurysms, and differentiation of mycotic from berry aneurysms is usually based on the location and size of the aneurysm. Mycotic aneurysms may heal following antibiotic therapy and not require surgical clipping. *(Annals of Neurology 27, p. 238, 1990; Ref. 1, p. 283)*

39. **A.** Noncontrast CT would show intracranial bleeding but would *not* show *small* mycotic aneurysms which may be the source of the hemorrhage. To demonstrate aneurysm, perform angiography. *(Annals Neurology 27, p. 238, 1990)*

13

DYSKINESIAS

True or False

1. _____ Kinetic tremor is characteristic of parkinsonism.

2. _____ Orthostatic hypotension is uncommon in parkinsonism.

3. _____ Dopamine loss from the substantia nigra results in parkinsonism.

4. _____ Deprenyl slows the pathological and chemical progression of parkinsonism as well as causing symptomatic improvement.

5. _____ Dopamine can accelerate neuronal death in parkinsonism.

6. _____ Parkinsonian tremor responds better to Sinemet than to anticholinergic medication.

7. _____ Oculogyric crisis is very often seen in idiopathic parkinsonism.

Multiple Choice

Choose the most appropriate response.

8. _____ Nonmotoric deficits in Parkinson disease include:

   A. Autonomic dysfunction
   B. Orthostatic hypotension
   C. Dementia
   D. Affective disorders
   E. All of the above

9. _____ Clinical findings in Parkinson's disease include:

   A. Stooped posture
   B. Retropulsion
   C. Festination
   D. Low-volume speech
   E. All of the above

10. _____ Sinemet is preferable to L-DOPA alone because of the following characteristics:

   A. Levodopa can cross the blood–brain barrier
   B. Dopamine does not cross the blood–brain barrier
   C. Can deliver lower levodopa dose with Sinemet than with L-DOPA alone
   D. Reduces systemic toxicity
   E. All of the above

11. _____ Long-term complications of dopaminergic agents include:

   A. Dyskinesias
   B. Dystonias
   C. End-of-dose deterioration
   D. On–off phenomenon
   E. All of the above

12. _____ The following surgical procedure may be effective in advanced parkinsonism:

   A. Thalamotomy
   B. Pallidotomy
   C. Fetal nigral transplant
   D. Adrenal medullary brain implant
   E. All of the above

13. _____ A 30-year-old attorney develops side-to-side rhythmical head shaking and difficulty speaking. What other neurological findings might be seen in this patient?

   A. Masklike facies
   B. Impaired postural reflexes
   C. Bradykinesia
   D. Kayser-Fleischer ring
   E. Difficulty using hands to bring cup to mouth

14. _____ Patients with Tourette syndrome may show these features:

   A. Parkinsonian features
   B. Obsessive-compulsive behavior
   C. Seizures
   D. Dementia
   E. Ataxia

15. _____ Neck dystonia may result from this medication:

A. Reglan
B. Tegretol
C. Phenobarbital
D. Deprenyl
E. Dilantin

16. _____ The following characteristics are true of patients with dystonia musculorum deformans:

A. Dystonia is usually initiated by activity
B. Disorder is hereditary and progressive
C. Dystonia is generalized
D. All of the above
E. None of the above

17. _____ One of the most important clinical differences between tardive dyskinesia and Huntington's disease is:

A. Gait is normal in tardive dyskinesia, whereas it is almost always abnormal in Huntington's disease
B. The rate and amplitude of dyskinesia are different in these two conditions
C. The pattern of dyskinesia is different in these two disorders
D. The muscle tone is different in these two disorders
E. Cognitive impairment is present only in Huntington's disease

18. _____ In the Westphal variant of Huntington's disease, the following is true:

A. Occurrence is rare before age 50
B. Patients have prominent dyskinesia
C. Patients appear rigid
D. Patients have no parkinsonian features
E. CT shows cerebellar abnormalities

19. _____ The following is true of oral-facial-lingual-masticatory dyskinesias:

A. 3–5% incidence in patients older than 65
B. May be precipitated by neuroleptics
C. Always progress and worsen in both distribution and severity of the dyskinesia
D. Are associated with mental change
E. Presenting finding in Parkinson disease

20. _____ The most prominent symptom of Shy-Drager syndrome is:

A. Progressive autonomic deficit
B. Cerebellar ataxia
C. Parkinsonism
D. Peripheral neuropathy
E. Dementia

21. _____ If a patient with suspected parkinsonian features shows no response to dopaminergic medication, consider this disorder as a possible alternative disorder.

A. Cortico-basal degeneration
B. Striato-nigral degeneration
C. Olivo-pontocerebellar degeneration
D. All of the above
E. None of the above

22. _____ The following is true of spasticity:

A. Due to injury involving corticospinal tract and anterior horn cell
B. Due to injury of corticospinal tract
C. Associated with cogwheel phenomena
D. Sometimes associated with flaccid weakness
E. Patients show other features consistent with Parkinson's disease

23. _____ This drug is effective in reducing spasticity:

A. Baclofen
B. L-DOPA
C. Methylphenidate
D. Phenytoin
E. Parlodel

24. _____ Akathisia may be a manifestation of:

A. Neuroleptic effect
B. Idiopathic parkinsonism
C. Chorea
D. Myoclonus
E. Athetosis

Answer based on the clinical history.

J.M. is a 48-year-old judge who notes tremor in his voice and deterioration in his handwriting. These symptoms are worse during periods of emotional stress. Examination shows side-to-side head and neck tremor and intention tremor of hands.

25. _____ The most likely diagnostic possibility is:

A. Essential tremor
B. Hyperthyroidism
C. Cerebellar neoplasm
D. Parkinsonism
E. Huntington's disease

26. _____ The most useful diagnostic test is:

   A. CT
   B. MRI
   C. EEG
   D. Chromosome studies
   E. Clinical observation

27. _____ If the patient were to have several alcoholic drinks before work, the tremor would most likely:

   A. Increase
   B. Decrease
   C. Not change
   D. Become generalized
   E. Interfere with walking

28. _____ Treatment of this type of tremor includes:

   A. Diazepam
   B. Lithium
   C. Depakote
   D. Phenytoin
   E. Cyclosporine

29. _____ If the patient were to die suddenly of unrelated myocardial infarction, brain autopsy findings referable to the tremor would include:

   A. Dopamine depletion in the substantia nigra
   B. Caudate atrophy
   C. Cerebellar atrophy
   D. Reduced brain catecholamine content
   E. No abnormalities

H.C. is a 52-year-old man who reports "shaking" in his right hand when he sits and watches television. He also notes difficulty utilizing tools and utensils. Examination shows 3-cps resting tremor in the right hand, mild bradykinesia, masklike facies, and postural instability.

30. _____ The most likely diagnosis is:

   A. Left basal ganglia infarct
   B. Left basal ganglia astrocytoma
   C. Left cerebellar metastases
   D. Parkinson's disease
   E. None of the above

31. _____ The most useful diagnostic study to establish the diagnosis would be:

   A. CT
   B. MRI
   C. PET
   D. SPECT
   E. None of the above

32. _____ If all studies are negative, the initial management strategy should be:

   A. High-dose Sinemet
   B. Low-dose Sinemet
   C. Artane
   D. Parlodel
   E. None of the above

33. _____ If the patient is treated with Sinemet and chorea develops in the arms and hands, the following medication adjustment should be made:

   A. Lower dose of Sinemet
   B. Increase dose of Sinemet
   C. Utilize Deprenyl
   D. Consider pallidotomy
   E. Add Artane

J.P. is a 38-year-old attorney who begins to act in a "bizarre" manner. One evening he goes to Bourbon Street and shoots three "enemies of the state." He is admitted to psychiatry service. He is psychotic with paranoid delusions, but the remainder of the neurological examination is normal. He responds well to Haldol and is maintained on this medication. One year later his Haldol dose is reduced. He develops arm fidgetiness and involuntary shoulder tics.

34. _____ The most likely diagnosis for the new symptoms which develop when the Haldol dose is reduced is:

   A. Parkinsonism
   B. Tardive dyskinesia
   C. Wilson's disease
   D. Alzheimer's's disease
   E. None of the above

35. _____ The most useful next diagnostic study would be:

   A. CT
   B. MRI
   C. EEG
   D. Serum ceruloplasmin
   E. Family history assessment

36. _____ If family history suggests neurological or psychiatric illness, the most likely diagnostic consideration would be:

   A. Huntington's disease
   B. Alzheimer's disease
   C. Parkinson's disease
   D. Schizophrenia
   E. Wilson's disease

37. _____ The most useful diagnostic study(ies) would be:

    A. Chromosome analysis
    B. PET
    C. CT
    D. MRI
    E. All of the above

A 48-year-old woman complains of right shoulder pain. This was diagnosed as "arthritis" and is being treated with aspirin. She has noted right-hand tremor when playing cards. Her brother died of Parkinson's disease. She becomes "sad" and has multiple crying episodes. Her appetite is poor and she has early morning awakenings. Examination shows right-sided resting tremor, hypomimia, decreased associated right arm movements when she walks.

38. _____ The most likely diagnosis is:

    A. Drug-induced parkinsonism
    B. Parkinson's disease and depression
    C. Huntington's disease
    D. Essential tremor
    E. Alzheimer's disease

39. _____ The most useful diagnostic study would be:

    A. CT
    B. MRI
    C. LP
    D. EEG
    E. None of the above

40. _____ Initial treatment should include:

    A. Elavil
    B. Cogentin
    C. Deprenyl
    D. Prozac
    E. None of the above

41. _____ The following combination should not be used:

    A. Deprenyl-Parnate
    B. Sinemet-Deprenyl
    C. Artane-Sinemet
    D. Sinemet-Parlodel
    E. Parlodel-Artane

A 60-year-old man develops memory loss and experiences visual hallucinations. He also has walking impairment, with slow, shuffling gait and postural instability. Treatment with Haldol improves the hallucinations but his gait worsens. Treatment with Sinemet does not improve his gait. He has increased hallucinations which cause agitation and confusion. Examination shows dementia, vertical gaze impairment, pseudobulbar palsy, bilateral Babinski signs, and rigidity.

42. _____ Diagnostic possibilities include:

    A. Alzheimer's disease
    B. Diffuse Lewy body disease
    C. Progressive supranuclear palsy
    D. All of the above
    E. None of the above

43. _____ Treatment should include:

    A. Sinemet-Clozapine
    B. Haldol-Sinemet
    C. Sinemet-Risperdal
    D. Artane-Haldol
    E. Sinemet-Cognex

44. _____ Definitive diagnosis is established by:

    A. CT
    B. MRI
    C. Neuropsychological testing
    D. EEG
    E. None of the above

45. _____ Extrapyramidal dysfunction in which of the following conditions responds to low-dose dopaminergic medication:

    A. Progressive supranuclear palsy
    B. Vascular parkinsonism
    C. Diffuse Lewy body disease
    D. Alzheimer's disease
    E. None of the above

46. _____ Diagnostic criteria for diffuse Lewy body disease include:

    A. Fluctuating cognitive impairment
    B. Hallucinations with paranoid content
    C. Extrapyramidal features and exaggerated neuroleptic sensitivity
    D. Gait disorder and frequent falls
    E. All of the above

RESPONSES AND EXPLANATIONS

1. **F.** Resting tremor at a rate of 3 cps which involves the patient's hands in a pill-rolling pattern is characteristic of parkinsonism. Kinetic intentional tremor is consistent with cerebellar dysfunction. *(Ref. 2, pp. 625–626; Ref. 4, pp. 242–243)*

2. **T.** In patients with parkinsonism-like features, the additional finding of orthostatic hypotension (which is a sign of autonomic dysfunction) suggests Shy-Drager syndrome. Also, remember that dopaminergic medication may cause this side effect. *(Ref. 2, p. 629)*

3. **T.** Parkinsonism results from dopamine deficiency, with loss of dopamine-producing cells in the substantia nigra. *(Ref. 2, p. 628)*

4. **T.** Based on results of several studies, selegiline (Deprenyl, Eldepryl), which is a selective monoamine oxidase B inhibitor, acts as a neuroprotective agent to reduce oxidative stress and prevent free-radical formation. It also causes *symptomatic* benefit by increasing synaptic dopamine. *(Ref. 2, p. 634)*

5. **F.** There is no convincing evidence that early treatment with Sinemet or other dopaminergic agents accelerates neuronal cell death. Dopaminergic agents should be initiated at low dose, then slowly and gradually increased to reduce functional motor disability. *(Mayo Clinic Proceedings 71, p. 659, 1996)*

6. **F.** For patients with resting tremor as the sole manifestation of parkinsonism, utilize anticholinergic medication (Artane, Cogentin). In some cases, *no* treatment may be necessary, because the resting tremor causes no functional motor impairment but is merely embarrassing for the patient. *(Ref. 2, p. 631)*

7. **F.** Oculogyric crisis is *uncommon* with *idiopathic* parkinsonism; however, this phenomenon is common in postencephalitic cases. It may also be seen in *drug-induced* parkinsonism. *(Ref. 1, pp. 714–715)*

8. **E.** Although classic symptoms involve motor and gait impairment (resting tremor, bradykinesia, rigidity), nonmotor dysfunction such as autonomic dysfunction and cognitive-behavioral features may occur. When these symptoms are prominent, consider alternative diagnostic possibilities, e.g,. Lewy body disease, Alzheimer's disease. *(Ref. 4, pp. 242–243)*

9. **E.** All the listed findings are characteristic of parkinsonism. Both speech (slow, monotonous, low volume) and writing (micrographia) are affected. Impaired postural reflexes may lead to frequent falls and result in orthopedic injuries including broken hip. *(Ref. 1, pp. 713–717)*

10. **E.** Levodopa may be used in combination with decarboxylase inhibitor (Sinemet) to cause fewer *systemic* (peripheral) side effects than levodopa alone. This allows use of a lower levodopa dose. Sinemet does not reduce *CNS* side effects. Dopamine does not cross the blood–brain barrier. *(Ref. 2, pp. 629–633)*

11. **E.** With long-term utilization of dopaminergic agents, all listed effects occur. It is possible that these effects result from disease progression rather than simply medication effect. Dyskinesias such as chorea may develop *early* if the dose of Sinemet is increased to high levels too rapidly. *(Ref. 2, pp. 629–633)*

12. **E.** All the listed surgical procedures have been tried in *medically intractable* Parkinson's disease. Pallidotomy is currently being utilized as the safest and most effective procedure. *(Ref. 1, pp. 722–723)*

13. **E.** Head movements are characteristic of essential tremor. This may also cause vocal and upper-extremity tremor. The latter may interfere with writing, utilizing tools and utensils, shaving, or bringing a cup to the mouth. Essential tremor does not effect the lower extremities. Remember this rule: *All that shakes is not parkinsonism.* Essential tremor is frequently mistaken for parkinsonism but it does *not* respond to dopaminergic agents. Kayser-Fleischer ring is characteristic of Wilson's disease, which may cause parkinsonian features or severe proximal upper-extremity tremor. *(Ref. 2, pp. 635–636)*

14. **B.** In Tourette syndrome, behavioral features including obsessive-compulsive disorder and attention-deficit-hyperactivity syndrome commonly accompany tics. *(Ref. 2, pp. 638–640)*

15. **A.** Reglan is an antiemetic agent frequently utilized in migraine patients. Reglan may cause neck dystonia, as do Compazine and Thorazine. Deprenyl is a selective MAO inhibitor which affects dopamine metabolism but does not usually cause dyskinesias. Dilantin and Tegretol may rarely cause tremor or asterixis at toxic levels. *(Ref. 2, pp. 646–649)*

16. **E.** This disorder occurs in children and adolescents. Clinical features include slow inversion and plantar flexion of the foot (equinovarus deformity). Dystonia becomes generalized to involve the upper extremities. At a later stage, posture become fixed, causing skeletal deformities. There are two genetic forms, autosomal recessive and dominant. *(Ref. 2, pp. 644–645)*

17. **E.** Cardinal features of HD are chorea and progressive cognitive-behavioral disorders. Based on clinical characteristics of motor abnormality of tardive dyskinesia, this may simulate HD. The family history and chromosomal studies may be

necessary to differentiate these two conditions. *(Ref. 2, pp. 637–638)*

18. **C.** In the Westphal (juvenile) variant of HD, patients may show muscle *rigidity;* whereas in adult HD patients, motor tone is *hypotonic. (Ref. 1, pp. 695–699)*

19. **B.** Neuroleptic medication may cause:
    a. Acute dystonic reaction
    b. Akathisia
    c. Parkinsonism
    d. Tardive dyskinesias (TD)
    TD consist of repetitive stereotyped movements which may resemble chorea. *Rarely*, they become severe enough to interfere with speaking, swallowing, or respiration. TD is most likely caused by high-potency neuroleptics. If detected early, reduction in dose or discontinuation of medication may cause movements to disappear. *(Ref. 1, pp. 733–736)*

20. **A.** In Shy-Drager syndrome, autonomic dysfunction is the major clinical feature in addition to parkinsonism. *(Ref. 1, pp. 720–721)*

21. **D.** More than 90% of patients with idiopathic PD initially respond to Sinemet. Failure to respond should suggest alternative degenerative neurological disorders. Since there is no neurodiagnostic test for PD, the diagnosis is clinical. *(Ref. 4, pp. 244–247)*

22. **B.** Spasticity is a state of muscle hypertonicity due to lesions involving the corticospinal or corticobulbar tracts. It is associated with increased deep tendon reflexes, positive Babinski sign, and motor impairment which includes weakness. It primarily involves antigravity muscles. In *rigidity*, there is *no* weakness or abnormal reflexes. *(Ref. 2, pp. 12, 141, 386)*

23. **A.** Spasticity is best treated with physical therapy, Baclofen, Dantrium, or muscle relaxant medication (Valium, Flexeril). *(Ref. 2, pp. 12, 141,386)*

24. **A.** Akathisia is motor restlessness. The patient feels unable to sit still. Manifestations include tapping of feet, body shifting, and body rocking. It is usually a side effect of neuroleptic medication. Motor restlessness may be seen as a manifestation of psychosis. It remits when antipsychotic medication is discontinued or may be reduced by anticholinergic medication. *(Ref. 1, pp. 733–736)*

25. **A.** This pattern is classic for "essential tremor." All dyskinesias worsen under emotional stress. This tremor can be precipitated by caffeine, fatigue, exercise, hyperthyroidism, medication (lithium, valproic acid, theophylline). This tremor never affects the legs. *(Ref. 2, pp. 640–641)*

26. **E.** This is a clinical diagnosis, and findings are so characteristic that no neurodiagnostic studies are necessary. *(Neurology 37, p. 1194, 1987; Ref. 2, pp. 640–641)*

27. **B.** This tremor is markedly reduced by the effects of alcohol. Some patients will self-medicate themselves with alcohol to ameliorate the disabling effect of tremor on activities of daily living. *(Ref. 1, pp. 712–713; Ref. 2, pp. 640–641)*

28. **A.** Medical treatment includes diazepam, mysoline, and beta-adrenergic blocking agents. All other listed drugs *exacerbate* the tremor. *(Ref. 1, pp. 712–713)*

29. **E.** Autopsy studies have shown no pathological changes; therefore this must be a neurotransmitter (neurochemical) abnormality. Some studies have shown increased incidence of PD developing in patients who initially present with essential tremor. *(Neurology 37, p. 1194, 1987)*

30. **D.** PD may begin as a unilateral, asymmetrical disorder; however, the postural instability and masklike facies indicate that this is a bilateral disorder and *not* due to a localized basal ganglia pathological lesion. If *all* the features were on the right side, this would suggest left-sided focal basal ganglia lesion. *(Ref. 4, pp. 242–243)*

31. **E.** Because of bilateral findings, idiopathic PD is the most likely diagnosis, and neurodiagnostic studies are unnecessary. *(Ref. 4, pp. 242–243; Ref. 5, pp. 8–12)*

32. **B.** Initiate treatment with the lowest dose of Sinemet and *gradually* increase the dose. There is no evidence that dopamine agonists (Parlodel) are more effective or safer treatment. Artane is most effective when tremor is the predominant symptom. Symptomatic treatment is indicated because the motor symptoms interfere with daily living activities. *(Neurology 40[suppl. 3], p. 1, 1990)*

33. **A.** The development of chorea indicates that the dose of dopaminergic medication is excessive and needs to be lowered. There is no difference in the incidence of CNS side effects between L-DOPA and Sinemet. *(Ref. 2, pp. 622–623)*

34. **E.** Cognitive-behavioral disturbances and chorea which develop in a 38-year-old man who has no prior psychiatric history suggests Huntington's disease. The abnormal movements do not involve the face; therefore tardive dyskinesia is unlikely. *(Ref. 2, pp. 637–638)*

35. **E.** HD is inherited as an autosomal dominant disorder; therefore a carefully obtained family history should be the next step. Be cognizant that the history may be negative, as some patients may die before they develop symptoms of HD. *(Ref. 1, pp. 695–699)*

36. **A.** If the family history is positive, HD is the most likely possibility; however, serum ceruloplasmin and slit-lamp eye exam (look for Kayser-Fleischer ring), looking for Wilson's disease, should be performed. *(Ref. 1, pp. 699–703)*

37. **E.** Chromosome 4 needs to be examined carefully for *DNA* (trinucleotide repeat) *expansion syndrome.* CT/MRI may show caudate atrophy, and PET may show caudate hypometabolism, even if the caudate shows no atrophy. *(Ref. 4, pp. 250–252)*

38. **B.** The initial symptom of right shoulder arthritis may actually be a manifestation of early PD. In this case, the "stiffness" due to PD rigidity may falsely simulate arthritis. Later, resting tremor develops, confirming the PD diagnosis. In addition, the patient has criteria for psychiatric diagnosis of major depression. *(Ref. 2, pp. 242–243)*

39. **E.** These are clinical diagnoses, and neurodiagnostic studies can be expected to show negative results. *(Ref. 2, pp. 242–243)*

40. **E.** It is possible that PD is the initial disorder and depression has developed secondary to PD. I suggest initiating treatment with Sinemet to obtain symptomatic relief of PD. I would not use Artane or Deprenyl, as they would not give adequate symptomatic relief of PD. *(Ref. 1, p. 728)*

41. **A.** It is probably unwise to utilize selective (Deprenyl) and nonselective (Parnate) MAO inhibitors in the same patient. All the other combinations would not cause dangerous drug interactions. *(Ref. 1, pp. 725–726)*

42. **C.** In PD, 90% of patients respond to dopaminergic medication; therefore failure to respond raises the possibility of an alternative diagnosis, e.g., progressive supranuclear palsy (PSP). The findings of vertical gaze impairment, Babinski signs, and pseudobulbar palsy are consistent with PSP. *(Ref. 1, pp. 722–726)*

43. **A.** To treat parkinsonian features, utilize Sinemet. Failure to respond confirms that this is not PD. Utilize Clozaril to treat behavioral symptoms, as this neuroleptic drug does *not* worsen PD, whereas Haldol worsens symptoms of PD. *(Ref. 1, pp. 721–726)*

44. **E.** Diagnosis can only be established by autopsy findings. *(Ref. 1, pp. 715–725)*

45. **E.** Parkinsonian features may be seen in all these listed conditions; however, response to any dopaminergic medication is poor. Only PD responds well to dopaminergic medication. *(Ref. 4, pp. 240–243)*

46. **E.** In diffuse Lewy body disease, patients show parkinsonian features plus prominent cognitive-behavioral disorders. *(Neurology 40, p. 1, 1990)*

14

PERIPHERAL NERVE AND MOTOR NEURON DISEASE

True or False

1. _____ In peripheral neuropathy, Babinski sign is likely to be plantar extensor.

2. _____ In patients with peripheral neuropathy, neurogenic bladder is an early and common clinical feature.

3. _____ A stocking-glove sensory pattern is characteristic of peripheral neuropathy and is not seen in other neurological disorders.

4. _____ In peripheral neuropathy, the "saddle" region shows early sensory disturbances.

Multiple Choice

Choose the most appropriate response.

5. _____ Patients with Guillain-Barré syndrome most commonly show:

   A. Proximal muscle weakness
   B. Absent sensation in feet and hands
   C. Bilateral facial weakness
   D. Absent deep tendon reflexes
   E. Bilateral Babinski signs

6. _____ The natural history of motor neuron disease includes:

   A. Slow initial progression and subsequent later stabilization of motor function
   B. Rapid early deterioration and subsequent stabilization of motor function
   C. Slow, insidious, progressive neurological deterioration of motor function
   D. Slow progression for several years, followed by sudden deterioration of motor function
   E. All of the above

7. _____ Effective therapy for acute inflammatory demyelinating polyneuropathy includes:

   A. Corticosteroids
   B. Plasma exchange
   C. Interferon
   D. None of the above
   E. All of the above

8. _____ The following is true of meralgia paresthetica:

   A. Characterized by anterolateral thigh dysaesthesia
   B. Due to entrapment of lateral femoral cutaneous nerve
   C. Etiologies include diabetes, tight-fitting garments
   D. All of the above
   E. None of the above

Matching

Match the unique clinical feature with the nerve disorder.

   A. Initially begins with hand numbness without leg symptoms
   B. Bilateral foot drop with accompanying orthopedic deformities in legs
   C. Numbness in specific limb regions; mutilated injured extremities; normal reflexes and proprioception sensation
   D. Autonomic dysfunction associated with mixed sensorimotor neuropathy
   E. Rapidly progressing distal extremity weakness which subsequently ascends to cranial nerve dysfunction

9. _____ Guillain-Barré syndrome

10. _____ Lepromatous neuropathy

11. _____ Diabetic neuropathy

12. _____ Charcot-Marie-Tooth syndrome

13. _____ Carpel tunnel syndrome

Match the clinical findings with the neurological condition.

A. Weakness of forearm flexion; biceps fasciculations; absent biceps reflex; pain and sensory loss in upper arm and radial forearm

B. Wasting and weakness of intrinsic hand muscles; widespread fasciculations; normal reflexes

C. Decreased sensation in stocking-glove distribution; positive Romberg sign; absent reflexes

D. Weakness and wasting of hands and feet with widespread fasciculations; hyperactive reflexes; bilateral Babinski signs

E. Scissoring gait; normal arm strength; normal sensation; bilateral Babinski signs; normal bladder function

14. _____ Primary lateral sclerosis

15. _____ Cervical radiculopathy

16. _____ Amyotrophic lateral sclerosis (ALS)

17. _____ Peripheral neuropathy

18. _____ Progressive muscular atrophy

Multiple Choice

Respond based on the clinical history.

L.G. is a 35-year-old professional baseball player. He notes difficulty holding his bat and is easily fatigued by the fifth inning of each game. Examination shows weakness of hand muscles, interossei wasting, and fasciculations in his forearm, calves, and tongue. Sensory exam is normal. He has bilateral plantar extensor responses.

19. _____ These findings can be best explained by:

A. Bilateral ulnar neuropathy
B. Subacute combined system disease
C. Cervical radiculopathy
D. Cervical myelopathy
E. ALS

20. _____ A high-yield diagnostic study in this patient would be:

A. EMG/NCV
B. Sural nerve biopsy
C. Spinal CT
D. Myelogram
E. Spinal MRI

21. _____ Appropriate ancillary studies after the diagnosis has been established include:

A. Cardiac stress test
B. Tensilon test

C. Pulmonary function studies
D. Cystometrogram
E. Neuropsychological tests

22. _____ Potential medical complications of this neurological disease include:

A. Aspiration pneumonia
B. Meningitis
C. Urinary tract infection
D. Cerebral infarction
E. Dementia

23. _____ Proven efficacious therapy for this disorder is:.

A. Thyrotrophin-stimulating hormone (TSH)
B. Neurotrophic growth factors
C. Antioxidant medication
D. Glutamate inhibitors
E. None of the above

24. _____ If the condition progresses, this might be expected to develop:

A. Dysarthria
B. Dysphagia
C. Facial paresis
D. Palatal weakness
E. All of the above

25. _____ Other neurological disturbances seen in ALS patients include:

A. Diplopia
B. Gaze paresis
C. Dementia
D. Hypoglossal atrophy
E. Sensory impairment in the limbs

RESPONSES AND EXPLANATIONS

1. **F.** Babinski sign indicates corticospinal tract dysfunction and therefore would not be positive in a lower motor neuron disorder, such as peripheral neuropathy. Babinski sign is positive only with motor cortex, subcortical (internal capsule), brainstem, or spinal cord dysfunction. *(Neurology 47, pp. 10–17, 1996; Ref. 2, pp. 34–35; Ref. 4, pp. 96–99)*

2. **F.** In patients with symptoms and signs of motor and sensory dysfunction involving the feet and legs (indicating lower lumbar and sacral distribution), bladder, bowel, and sexual dysfunction suggest spinal cord (myelopathy) or multiple root (radiculopathy) involvement. Polyneuropathy rarely causes neurogenic bladder, although certain neuropathies have autonomic components resulting in neurogenic bladder and/or bowel dysfunction. As a general rule, if neurogenic bladder is present, think spinal pathology and perform spinal imaging studies. *(Ref. 4, pp. 6–7, 24–29)*

3. **F.** Stocking-glove sensory impairment may be seen with peripheral neuropathy but is also seen in conversion reactions. In neuropathy, sensory loss in the legs extends quite proximally before the hands are affected. Also, in neuropathy, there is gradual *grading* or reduction of sensory impairment in the proximal direction, e.g., most severe in the toes, less severe in the legs, and least in the thighs; whereas in conversion reaction, there is *sharp cutoff* from abnormal to normal regions, usually at mid-calf and mid-forearm level. *(Ref. 2, pp. 157–164; Ref. 4, pp. 92–95)*

4. **F.** In neuropathy, distal involvement occurs in the longest nerves initially. The saddle (perineal) region is supplied by *short* nerves, but these are derived by *distal* sacral roots (S-2, S-3, S-4). Sacral involvement is invariably associated with autonomic (bowel, bladder, sexual) dysfunction, and this disturbance suggests spinal lesion. *(Ref. 2, pp. 161–162, 602–603; Ref. 4, pp. 6–7)*

5. **D.** In acute ascending polyneuropathy of Guillain-Barré type (GBS), there is initial *distal* weakness, usually with preserved sensation (although there may be sensory *symptoms*). Deep tendon reflexes are *invariably* absent or markedly decreased. Weakness *may* sometimes extend to cranial nerves, causing facial immobility, dysphagia, or respiratory disturbances. With polyneuropathy, Babinski signs are *never* positive. *(Ref. 1, pp. 657–660; Ref. 2, pp. 476–479)*

6. **C.** Motor neuron disease, of which one form is amyotrophic lateral sclerosis, is a degenerative disorder affecting the upper and lower motor neurons. As with this and other degenerative conditions, there is *slow,* inexorable progression, usually *without* periods of stabilization or improvement. *(Ref. 1, pp. 744–748; Ref. 4, pp. 12–13)*

7. **B.** In GBS, neurological improvement can be hastened by plasma exchanges (plasmapheresis). Effective therapy may also include intravenous immunoglobulins but not interferon (this is effective for multiple sclerosis). Corticosteroids have been utilized for GBS, but evidence suggests that they may *prolong* clinical course and *increase* pulmonary complications. There is *no* evidence that they improve outcome. Corticosteroids may also cause serious complications, including GI bleeding, mood swings and psychoses, hypertension, osteoporosis, cataracts, and glaucoma. *(Ref. 1, pp. 657–660; Ref. 2, pp. 476–479)*

8. **D.** All statements are true. When this condition occurs, carefully evaluate the patient for diabetes mellitus. The intense paresthesias (which represents deafferentation pain) may respond to treatment with amitriptyline. *(Ref. 2, pp. 157–165, 171–175)*

9. **E**
10. **C**
11. **D**
12. **B**
13. **A**

9–13. Carpel tunnel syndrome is a *focal* compressive neuropathy which indicates dysfunction of the median nerve (as it passes through the transverse carpal ligament at the wrist). Charcot-Marie-Tooth is congenital neuropathy in which there is marked wasting of the feet (stork-limb deformity) with accompanying orthopedic conditions (pes cavus, hammer toes, scoliosis). Leprosy causes involvement of cutaneous and peripheral nerves. Cutaneous sensations (temperature, pain, light touch) are impaired but deep sensation (position and vibration) are preserved. Associated arthropathy and bone resorption (with loss of digits) frequently occurs. Diabetes mellitus is the most common neuropathy that causes autonomic nerve dysfunction. Very careful normoglycemic control delays onset of neuropathy, and neuropathy may be reversed by pancreatic transplant. GBS is a para-infectious demyelinating neuropathy which progresses *rapidly* and may ascend to involve the diaphragm, causing respiratory dysfunction, and the lower cranial nerves. *(Ref. 1, pp. 648–660; Ref. 2, pp. 163, 467)*

14. **E**
15. **A**
16. **D**
17. **C**
18. **B**

14–18. Cervical radiculopathy causes motor, sensory, and reflex disturbances *localized* to a specific level, e.g., C-5, C-6, or

C-7, due to nerve root impingement by a herniated cervical disk. Fasciculations are most commonly seen with anterior horn cell disease but *may* be seen in localized pattern with radiculopathy. Progressive muscular atrophy is a form of motor neuron disease in which there is *only* lower motor neuron findings. Weakness, wasting, and fasciculations without sensory disturbances and the presence of normal reflexes exclude cervical radiculopathy or myelopathy. Peripheral neuropathy causes proprioceptive loss which may result in positive Romberg sign. Absent reflexes are an early finding of neuropathy. In ALS, there are both upper and lower motor neuron signs with no sensory or autonomic disturbances. In primary lateral sclerosis, there are only upper motor neuron signs. These most predominantly involve the legs (paraparesis). This results in bilateral circumducting gait due to weakness and spasticity (scissoring). There are positive Babinski signs, consistent with corticospinal tract dysfunction. Lack of sensory disturbances and bladder dysfunction exclude spinal cord lesions (myelopathy). *(Ref. 1, pp. 744–748; Ref. 2, pp. 488–492; Ref. 4, pp. 24–25, 224–225)*

19. **E.** The upper and lower motor neuron signs with normal sensation indicate ALS as the most likely diagnosis. Also, tongue fasciculations exclude spinal lesion. *(Ref. 2, pp. 488–492; Ref. 4, pp. 224–225)*

20. **A.** In ALS, nerve conduction velocity is normal and electromyogram shows denervation muscle potentials. Since the sural nerve has *only* a sensory component, biopsy would be normal in motor neuron disease. Since clinical features are *widespread,* it is unlikely that they are caused by a *localized* spinal cord lesion. In some cases, the clinical features of ALS are localized and do not initially include bulbar features; therefore neuro-imaging studies might be warranted to exclude spinal lesions. *(Ref. 4, pp. 224–225)*

21. **C.** Patients with ALS die of pulmonary complications. It is important to monitor pulmonary function. Patients with ALS do not develop cognitive impairment; however, depression is not an unexpected feature of this uniformly fatal illness. Remember that as weakness worsens, patients report "fatigue," but with all the other clinical features indicating ALS, there is nothing to suggest myasthenia as an alternative diagnosis even though "fatigue" is the most prominent feature of myasthenia; therefore, the Tensilon test is not necessary. *(Ref. 1, pp. 744–748)*

22. **A.** In patients with bulbar and pseudobulbar palsy, swallowing is impaired, resulting in aspiration pneumonia. Drooling of saliva is another complicating feature of ALS. *(Ref. 1, pp. 746–747)*

23. **E.** At present, there is no proven effective therapy. Use of TSH *may* transiently improve motor function. Current research has focused on the role of excitatory neurotransmitters such as glutamate in pathogenesis of ALS as well as on role of oxidative stress with possible value of MAD inhibitor. Use of glutamate receptor blockers may be effective in slowing the progression of motor weakness. Riluzole has been utilized to slow the course of motor neuron disease. Use of neurotrophic growth factors has not been shown to be effective, but clinical trials are ongoing. *(Neurology 47[suppl 2], pp. 117–126; Lancet 348, p. 795, 1991)*

24. **E.** As ALS progresses, there is bulbar dysfunction which leads to all the listed motor disturbances. *(Ref. 1, pp. 746–747)*

25. **D.** In patients suspected of having ALS, observe intrinsic tongue muscles. There is weakness of tongue (hypoglossal) muscles with fasciculations and atrophy. Learn to observe the tongue on the floor of the mouth because some normals will have fasciculations when the tongue is protruded. Eye movements are not affected, and cognition remains normal. *(Ref. 1, pp. 744–748; Ref. 2, pp. 488–492)*

15

MUSCLE AND GAIT DISORDERS

True or False

1. _____ All patients who complain of myalgias have poly-myositis.

2. _____ Muscular dystrophy is an inherited form of myopathy in which weakness usually worsens as the patient gets older.

3. _____ Patients with myopathy usually initially complain of difficulty arising from a chair or difficulty climbing steps.

4. _____ In early polymyositis, deep tendon reflexes are diminished.

5. _____ Fasciculations are characteristically seen in patients with myopathy.

6. _____ In parkinsonian patients with impaired postural reflexes, they characteristically fall "en bloc."

7. _____ Back-kneeing is due to weakness of the thigh muscles and poor knee stabilization; waddling gait is due to hip girdle muscle weakness.

8. _____ Patients with Friedreich's ataxia usually have positive Romberg sign.

9. _____ A broad-based unsteady base and station from which the patient falls to either side is consistent with cerebellar disturbance.

Multiple Choice

Choose the the most correct response.

10. _____ This enzyme is most commonly elevated in carriers of Duchenne muscular dystrophy.

    A. SGOT
    B. SGPT
    C. LDH
    D. CPK
    E. None of the above

11. _____ In patients with myasthenia gravis (MG), the following is the best predictor of a probable "mild" or "benign" course:

    A. Ptosis as only clinical feature for 7 years after diagnosis of MG has been established
    B. Presence of thymic hyperplasia in tissue obtained at thymectomy
    C. Low titer of acetylcholine receptor antibody
    D. All of the above
    E. None of the above

12. _____ In patients with myasthenic *syndrome,* autonomic nervous system disturbances and muscle weakness are due to:

    A. Postsynaptic muscarinic blockade
    B. Presynaptic acetylcholine receptor blockade
    C. Postsynaptic nicotine receptor blockade
    D. All of the above
    E. None of the above

13. _____ Fatigue is characteristic of this disorder:

    A. Myasthenia gravis
    B. Multiple sclerosis
    C. Chronic fatigue syndrome
    D. Motor neuron disease
    E. All of the above

14. _____ Myasthenia gravis frequently initially involves muscles in this region:

    A. Oropharynx
    B. Shoulder muscles
    C. Girdle muscles
    D. Hand muscles
    E. Extraocular and levator palpebral muscles

15. _____ Medications which should be avoided in myasthenia gravis patients include:

    A. Penicillamine
    B. Kanamycin
    C. Streptomycin
    D. Neomycin
    E. All of the above

16. _____ In myasthenic gravis workup, the physician should order these studies:

   A. MRI brain, MRI chest, EMG, anti-AChR titer
   B. MRI chest, EMG, anti-AChR titer
   C. MRI brain, EMG, anti-AChR titer
   D. None of the above
   E. All of the above

17. _____ All of the following are seen in patients with polymyositis, *except:*

   A. Weakness, and sometimes pain, principally involving girdle muscles
   B. An accompanying occult malignancy
   C. Muscle biopsy showing muscle fiber necrosis with inflammatory infiltrates consisting of lymphocytes and plasma cells
   D. EMG showing myopathic potentials
   E. Swallowing function may be impaired

18. _____ All of the following are disorders of the neuromuscular junction, *except:*

   A. Myasthenia gravis (MG)
   B. Eaton-Lambert syndrome
   C. Botulism
   D. ALS
   E. Neonatal myasthenia gravis

Matching

Match the clinical features with the disorder.

   A. Occurs in males only; patients rarely develop the capacity to walk normally; death due to heart failure
   B. Asymmetrical upper-extremity muscle weakness sparing the leg muscles; smile is asymmetrical
   C. Symmetrical proximal arm and leg weakness; inherited as autosomal recessive
   D. Weakness involves distal muscles; hands are stiff; cataracts and frontal balding occur
   E. Inherited as sex-linked recessive; calf pseudohypertrophy develops; ambulation possible even at age 20

19. _____ Becker dystrophy

20. _____ Limb-girdle dystrophy

21. _____ Facio-scapulohumeral dystrophy

22. _____ Myotonic dystrophy

23. _____ Duchenne dystrophy

Multiple Choice

Respond based on the clinical history.

A 40-year-old man develops diplopia, right eyelid drooping, and neck swelling. Resting pulse rate is 110 and he is anxious and diaphoretic. Eyelid drooping is not present when the patient awakens but develops and worsens during the morning. The patient has proptosis.

24. _____ The most likely diagnosis is:

   A. Myasthenia gravis
   B. Myasthenic syndrome
   C. Multiple sclerosis (MS)
   D. Hyperthyroidism
   E. A and D

25. _____ Which test would most likely establish the cause of the patient's symptoms?

   A. Single-fiber EMG
   B. Edrophonium test
   C. Acetylcholine receptor antibody
   D. Repetitive nerve stimulation
   E. All of the above

A 30-year-old attorney complains of weakness, muscle aches, and fatigue. Fatigues becomes so severe that he gives up his legal practice and goes on medical disability. Neurological examination is completely normal, including repetitive exercise testing.

26. _____ The most likely diagnosis is:

   A. Multiple sclerosis (MS)
   B. Myasthenia gravis (MG)
   C. Hyperthyroidism
   D. Briquet syndrome
   E. Chronic fatigue syndrome

27. _____ The following diagnostic test is most likely to show an abnormality:

   A. MRI brain
   B. EMG
   C. LP
   D. Tensilon test
   E. None of the above

28. _____ A diagnosis of clinical MS is unlikely because:

   A. Eye movements are normal
   B. Examination is normal
   C. Optic atrophy is not present
   D. Lhermitte sign is negative
   E. All of the above

RESPONSES AND EXPLANATIONS

1. **F.** Myalgias are aches and pains in muscles. These are subjective symptoms which may occur with many musculo-skeletal and rheumatological disorders, e.g., polymyalgia rheumatica. In polymyositis, patients complain of myalgias and muscle tenderness when muscles are palpated, and there is accompanying proximal muscle weakness. *(Ref. 4, pp. 56–57)*

2. **T.** Muscular dystrophy is an inherited primary muscle disease (myopathy). In this disorder, muscle does not form normally; therefore muscle dysfunction (weakness) worsens with time. In the most severe form of muscle dystrophy (Duchenne), both skeletal and cardiac muscle are involved. These patients never walk normally and are confined to a wheelchair early in life. They may die of cardiac decompensation. *(Ref. 1, pp. 768–780; Ref. 2, pp. 507–510)*

3. **T.** For undetermined factors, primary muscle disease (myopathy) initially involves proximal muscles and primary nerve disease (peripheral neuropathy, anterior horn cell) initially involves distal muscles. In myopathy, proximal weakness causes difficulty arising from the floor or a chair, and it may be difficult for the patient to lift objects (due to proximal shoulder girdle muscle weakness). Patients with primary nerve disease may trip while walking, due to foot-ankle (distal) weakness and instability. They may experience difficulty opening jars and bottles, due to hand weakness. *(Ref. 4, pp. 38–39)*

4. **F.** In early stages of neuropathy, reflexes are diminished due to *afferent* (sensory) pathway disturbances. In myopathy, reflexes are preserved until late; whereas in ALS, reflexes are *increased* due to the upper motor neuron component. *(Ref. 1, pp. 648–650)*

5. **F.** Fasciculations are characteristic of anterior horn cell disease; their presence indicates muscle denervation. They may also be seen in *localized* pattern in radiculopathies (cervical, thoracic, lumbar). When seen in pathological conditions, fasciculations are accompanied by muscle wasting. Fasciculations may *also* be seen in normals; however, normals have *no* other accompanying neurological disturbances. *(Ref. 4, pp. 54–55)*

6. **T.** In parkinsonism, there is impairment of postural reflexes, which causes frequent falls. This is tested by observing the patient attempt to regain balance when rapid destabilizing force (push) is applied to the sternum. When this is done, a normal subject rapidly regains balance; whereas a parkinsonian patient falls like a block of wood ("en bloc") and makes no effort to "right" himself without falling. The impaired postural reflexes may cause Parkinson's patients with accompanying "soft" (osteoporotic) bones to fall and break hip bones. *(Ref. 1, pp. 51–55)*

7. **T.** In patients with myopathies, there is weakness of pelvic girdle muscles such that there is waddling (broad-based) gait with back-kneeing due to thigh muscle weakness resulting in poor knee stabilization. *(Ref. 1, pp. 51–55; Ref. 2, pp. 143–147)*

8. **T.** In Friedreich's ataxia, gait ataxia is due to a combination of cerebellar *and* proprioceptive impairment. Due to proprioceptive impairment, Romberg sign is positive and some patients may even be unable to sit in a chair due to trunkal instability due to cerebellar dysfunction. *(Ref. 1, pp. 686–688; Ref. 2, pp. 461–462)*

9. **T.** In gait ataxia due to cerebellar disturbance, gait is clumsy and awkward. There is broad-based stance and posture; patient cannot perform tandem gait (heel to heel). Patient walks as if drunk and veers to either side. Gait is most commonly affected with midline vermal cerebellar disorders. *(Ref. 1, pp. 51–55; Ref. 2, pp. 146–151)*

10. **D.** Creatine kinase (CK) is present in highest concentration in skeletal and cardiac muscle. With muscle disease, this sarcoplasmic enzyme is released into the serum. Highest levels are seen in Duchenne dystrophy, polymyositis, and myoglobinuria. CK may be *slightly* elevated in neurogenic disease. In muscle disease, other sarcoplasmic enzymes (SGOT, SGPT, LDH) are also elevated. In *carriers* of Duchenne dystrophy, females who *carry* the gene may have isolated mild muscle weakness, calf pseudohypertrophy, and elevated serum CK. *(Ref. 1, pp. 97–99, 768–80)*

11. **A.** MG may remain as localized ocular muscle weakness or may become generalized to involve the limbs and bulbar muscles. If it is generalized, respiratory involvement may occur; however, respiratory disturbance does *not* occur in ocular MG. The most severe course of MG occurs within 7 years of onset; therefore, if the disease remains localized to the ocular muscle for 7 years, the course is likely to remain benign. There is no correlation of clinical severity with level of acetylcholine receptor antibody titer. *(Ref. 1, pp. 754–760; Ref. 2, pp. 526–535)*

12. **B.** In Eaton-Lambert syndrome, there is autoimmune disorder involving peripheral cholinergic synapses. There is reduced release of acetylcholine at *nicotinic* and *muscarinic* sites due to antibodies directed against voltage-gated calcium channels. This involves presynaptic acetylcholine receptor function. Symptoms include proximal limb weakness, reduced knee and ankle reflexes, dry mouth, paresthesias, impotence, and reduced sweating (hypohidrosis). Treatment includes drugs which enhance acetylcholine release, e.g., guanidine. *(Ref. 1, pp. 761–762; Ref. 2, pp. 526–535)*

13. **E.** Patients with muscle weakness of any etiology may complain that they tire or fatigue easily. In patients with fatigue due to neurological illness, neurological examination *always* shows abnormalities, and weakness is demonstrated with manual muscle testing. If clinical examination is normal, the cause of weakness and fatigue is *not* likely to be primary neurological illness. *(Ref. 4, pp. 44–45)*

14. **E.** In MG, ptosis and diplopia due to extraocular muscle involvement may be the initial symptoms. A defect in neuromuscular transmission may cause fluctuations in severity of symptoms (remissions, exacerbations). *(Ref. 1, pp. 754–760)*

15. **E.** Aminoglycosides (neomycin, streptomycin, kanamycin) or polypeptide antibiotics (polymyxin) cause neuromuscular transmission blockade. They should be avoided in myasthenic patients. D-penicillamine is used for rheumatoid arthritis and Wilson's disease and may cause drug-induced myasthenia and polymyositis. *(Ref. 1, pp. 761–763)*

16. **B.** In MG patients, antibodies to AChR are found in 90% of affected patients. They may be *absent* in ocular MG but are invariably present in generalized MG. The thymus appears enlarged in 70%, and thymus gland histology shows germinal hyperplasia. In 10% of cases, thymoma is present. CT and MRI of mediastinum are the most sensitive studies to detect thymus enlargement. Since MG does not cause CNS pathology, *brain* CT or MRI would not be expected to show an abnormality. EMG would show progressively *decremental* response of muscle action potential elicited by repetitive nerve stimulation. *(Ref. 1, p. 754)*

17. **B.** Polymyositis is an autoimmune disease due to altered *cellular* immunity, as contrasted to dermatomyositis, which is due to *antibody* abnormalities. Both cause proximal muscle weakness. EMG shows "myopathic" features and there are elevated CK levels in the serum. The definitive diagnosis of polymyositis is established by muscle biopsy findings showing muscle necrosis and regeneration with infiltration of muscle by CD8+ T-lymphocytes. There is *no* evidence of vasculitis within the muscle. Arthralgia, myalgia, and Raynaud phenomena may be present, but other collagen vascular diseases do not usually occur in patients with polymyositis. If skin rash is present in a patient with proximal muscle weakness, consider dermatomyositis; diagnosis is established by muscle (showing endothelial hyperplasia of intramuscular blood vessels) and skin biopsy. Polymyositis is *not* dermatomyositis minus the skin rash. Dermatomyositis in adults is frequently associated with occult neoplasm, but this is *not* true of polymositis. *(Ref. 1, pp. 798–802)*

18. **D.** All listed disorders involve defective neuromuscular transmission except ALS, which is a degenerative disorder of anterior horn cells. Botulinum toxin blocks nicotinic (muscle) and muscarinic (autonomic parasympathetic) cholinergic release. This may lead to respiratory paralysis. Weakness may be reversed by guanidine. *(Ref. 1, p. 763)*

19. **E**

20. **C**

21. **B**

22. **D**

23. **A**

19–23. Duchenne muscular dystrophy is an X-linked disorder due to mutation in the dystrophin gene at Xp21. It occurs in *males* only, with onset in *childhood,* initially involving the *pelvic* muscles, and there is usually calf muscle *pseudohypertrophy. Contractures* may develop in wasted muscles. Fascioscapulohumeral muscle dystrophy is an autosomal dominant disorder. It occurs in patients of either sex. Initial weakness is in the shoulder girdle muscles, and facial muscles are always involved. Legs are *not* weak. Limb-girdle dystrophy is inherited as autosomal recessive. Onset occurs during adolescence. There is symmetrical pelvic girdle and shoulder weakness. The course is that of slow progression of muscle weakness. Myotonic muscular dystrophy is an autosomal dominant *multisystem* disease. Features include cataracts, endocrine symptoms, and cardiac dysfunction. Cranial muscles are affected. Myotonia (failure to relax) is a characteristic feature. Becker dystrophy is a dystrophin disorder similar to Duchenne but with later age of onset and much slower progression; it causes less disability. *(Ref. 1, pp. 768–780)*

24. **E.** Both hyperthyroidism and MG may cause extraocular muscle involvement. The systemic signs in this patient suggest hyperthyroidism. The presence of proptosis would also be consistent with hyperthyroidism. Five to 10% of MG patients have associated hyperthyroidism because both conditions are immune mediated. Extraocular muscle dysfunction causing diplopia may be restrictive in dysthyroid ophthalmopathy or due to neuromuscular transmission defect in MG. The presence of prominent fatigue suggests that muscle weakness (ptosis) is due to MG rather than hyperthyroidism, but this fatigue could be due to either condition. *(Ref. 2, pp. 684–685)*

25. **E.** All pharmacological and electrophysiological tests may be utilized to determine if there is neuromuscular transmission defect due to MG. *(Ref. 1, pp. 754–757)*

26. **E.** If the patient has normal neurological examination and no evidence of muscle weakness on muscle testing, it is unlikely that there is clinical MG or MS. The patient has no systemic signs of hyperthyroidism; therefore that is unlikely to be the cause of the fatigue; however, laboratory studies for thyroid dysfunction *must* be performed to exclude this disorder. Briquet syndrome (conversion reaction) is a possibility, but the clinical features fit best with chronic fatigue syndrome (CFS). *(Ref. 1, p. 48; Ref. 2, p. 718; Ref. 4, pp. 44–45)*

27. **E.** With normal clinical neurological exam, it is unlikely that any tests would show an abnormality, but they should be done to exclude the *remote* possibility of a causal neurological condition. CFS represents a diagnosis of *exclusion* based on characteristic clinical features and negative diagnostic tests. (Ref. 2, p. 718)

28. **B.** In MS, optic neuritis may cause optic atrophy; spinal cord disorder could cause Lhermitte sign; brainstem (median longitudinal fasciculus) involvement could cause abnormal eye movements. In clinically symptomatic MS, however, the neurological examination can *never* be completely normal. Remember, there are rare patients who have pathological evidence of MG (found at autopsy) who never had clinical symptoms during life. *(Ref. 1, pp. 811–815)*

16

TRAUMATIC DISORDERS INCLUDING HEAD INJURIES

True or False

1. _____ Patients with carpal tunnel syndrome may experience tingling sensation over the fourth and fifth fingers, have weakness of thumb flexion, and show positive Tinel sign.

2. _____ A "lucid interval" is seen most commonly in patients who develop epidural hematoma. It may also be seen in patients with subdural hematoma or cerebral contusions.

3. _____ Neurological sequelae to head injury is unlikely unless there has been an initial loss of consciousness or amnesia for the event.

4. _____ Concussion and contusion are caused by diffuse axonal shearing injury.

5. _____ Basilar skull fractures may cause cranial nerve and hypothalamic-pituitary injury.

6. _____ Skull fractures developing across the middle meningeal artery groove are frequently associated with epidural hematomas.

7. _____ Following cerebral contusion, gliosis may develop at the injury site, and gliosis may lead to posttraumatic epilepsy.

8. _____ Subdural hematoma usually results from tearing of bridging cerebral veins.

9. _____ Boxers may develop dementia and parkinsonian features due to effects of head injury.

10. _____ As consequence of depressed skull fracture, a fragment of fractured bone is pushed inward, injuring underlying brain and possibly tearing the dura.

11. _____ In head injuries in which the patient experiences prolonged loss of consciousness but CT shows no focal brain injury, there is likely to be diffuse axonal shearing injury.

12. _____ In posttraumatic brain swelling, there may be both cerebral edema and abnormal vasodilatation.

13. _____ Traumatic brain contusions are frequently found in the basal ganglia and thalamus.

14. _____ Based on characteristic shape and location, CT findings can accurately differentiate epidural from subdural hematoma.

15. _____ All subdural hematomas must be surgically evacuated or neurological deficit will worsen.

16. _____ An abnormal collection of CSF located in subdural space is defined as subdural hygroma.

17. _____ Trauma to the carotid artery may cause carotid-cavernous fistula.

Multiple Choice

Respond based on the clinical history.

One week following a football-related head and neck injury, J.M. complains of right-sided neck pain and supraorbital headache. He is treated with acetaminophen with no improvement. Three days later, he awakens unable to move his right arm. Examination shows right hemiplegia and left-sided Horner syndrome.

18. _____ The most likely diagnosis is:

   A. Epidural hematoma
   B. Subdural hematoma
   C. Subarachnoid hemorrhage
   D. Carotid artery dissection
   E. Diffuse axonal shearing injury

19. _____ The initial diagnostic study should be:

   A. LP
   B. Skull radiogram
   C. CT
   D. MRI
   E. EEG

20. _____ The next diagnostic study should be:

A. Carotid duplex Doppler ultrasound
B. Cerebral angiogram
C. Sella tomograms
D. Magnetic resonance angiogram (MRA)
E. B and D

21. _____ Treatment for this trauma-related disorder should include:

A. Anticoagulation
B. Thrombolytic agents
C. Carotid endarterectomy
D. Carotid angioplasty
E. None of the above

True or False

Respond based on the clinical history.

Minnie Jismus was participating in gymnastics routine at cheerleading camp when she tumbled from the pyramid. No one was able to see whether she struck her head. She immediately complained of headache and dizziness. She was helped to a chair, but had to lie down due to generalized weakness. After vomiting once, she was taken to the emergency department. Upon examination, Minnie's mental status was normal, except that she appeared somewhat drowsy and complained of right-sided headache and nausea. The rest of the exam was normal, with no signs of papilledema, and her neck could be flexed forward without limitation.

22. _____ Even though Minnie's exam is nonfocal, she could have suffered a vascular event.

23. _____ Minnie is having her first migraine.

24. _____ Minnie must have a CT or MRI immediately.

25. _____ Minnie must have a lumbar puncture immediately.

Multiple Choice

Respond based on the clinical history.

J.J. is a 20-year-old college student who is attacked and beaten on Bourbon Street after leaving a brothel. He is lethargic, with evidence of ecchymoses around his eye and behind his right ear. Examination shows left facial weakness and left lateral rectus paresis.

26. _____ The most likely diagnosis is:

A. Basilar skull fracture
B. Cerebral concussion
C. Cerebral contusion
D. Cerebral laceration
E. White matter shearing injury

27. _____ The initial diagnostic study should be:

A. Skull radiogram
B. EEG
C. LP
D. CT
E. MRI

28. _____ A potential complication of this condition would include:

A. Rhinorrhea
B. Seizures
C. Syncope
D. Korsakoff syndrome
E. Dementia

29. _____ Five days later, J.J. develops headache and becomes febrile. Which diagnosis is most likely?

A. Meningitis
B. Subdural hematoma
C. Epidural hematoma
D. Delayed intracerebral hematoma
E. Traumatic subarachnoid hemorrhage

30. _____ Which cranial nerve dysfunction is most likely as a sequela to this type of injury?

A. Olfactory
B. Optic
C. Acoustic
D. Glossopharyngeal
E. Hypoglossal

31. _____ In a patient with basilar skull fracture, the following clinical finding(s) may develop:

A. Anosmia
B. Battle sign
C. Raccoon eyes
D. Rhinorrhea
E. All of the above

P.T. is an 8-year-old boy who falls off a playground swing and hits his head on the ground. He is unconscious for 2 min and has no memory of being on the swing before the accident. Exam is normal, including mental state.

32. _____ The most likely diagnosis based on the clinical features described is:

A. Cerebral concussion
B. Cerebral contusion
C. Epidural hematoma
D. Subdural hematoma
E. None of the above

33. _____ Management should include:

A. Observe carefully for 24 hr
B. Corticosteroids
C. Skull radiogram
D. CT
E. MRI

34. _____ Two hours later, P.T. complains of headache and vomits. Exam shows left dilated pupil and right hemiparesis. The most likely diagnosis is:

A. Right-sided epidural hematoma
B. Left-sided epidural hematoma
C. Left-sided subdural hematoma
D. Left-sided cerebral contusion
E. Left-sided intracerebral hematoma

35. _____ Management should include:

A. Hyperventilation
B. Mannitol
C. Immediate CT
D. Neurosurgical intervention
E. All of the above

RESPONSES AND EXPLANATIONS

1. **F.** In CTS, pain in the hand and wrist are expected findings. Sensory disturbances involve the thumb, index, and middle finger, which are median nerve innervated; the ulnar portion of the fourth and the entire fifth finger are ulnar innervated. Thumb flexion is median innervated but intrinsic hand muscles are ulnar innervated. Tinel sign is a general term referring to paresthesias evoked when palpating or percussing over a demyelinated nerve, e.g., the median nerve at the wrist, the ulnar nerve at the elbow. *(Ref. 2, pp. 163, 467; Ref. 4, pp. 216–218)*

2. **T.** "Lucid interval" refers to the time period after the patient recovers from concussive injury and before neurological condition deteriorates due to mass effect and intracranial hypertension secondary to trauma-induced mass lesion. The term "lucid interval" is most commonly seen with epidural hematoma but can occur with *any* trauma-induced lesion, e.g., subdural hematoma, cerebral contusion. *(Ref. 1, pp. 426–428; Ref. 2, pp. 366–367)*

3. **T.** Neurobehavioral sequelae to head injury are *unlikely* (but not impossible) if impairment of consciousness (dazed, stunned, confused) and/or memory loss (retro- or antegrade amnesia) do not occur. Following *head* injury, patients who have an initial Glasgow coma scale of 15 are unlikely to have suffered traumatic *brain* injury. *(Ref. 2, pp. 356–358)*

4. **F.** In concussion, CT/MRI show no abnormality, and the underlying pathological lesion may be a form of diffuse axonal shearing; however, autopsy studies from patients with concussion are extremely limited, as almost all patients survive. In contusion, there is tissue edema, necrosis, and hemorrhage; these are usually readily detected by CT/MRI. *(Ref. 1, p. 418; Ref. 2, pp. 356–362)*

5. **T.** Cranial nerves are anchored to the skull base and exit through individual foramina. The olfactory, optic, abducens, facial, and acoustic-vestibular are most frequently injured by trauma. Since the hypothalamus and pituitary are located at the skull base, endocrine disturbances including water-electrolyte disturbances may occur with skull base injuries. *(Ref. 1, p. 436)*

6. **T.** In more than 50% of patients with EDH, the fracture crosses the middle meningeal artery groove and bleeding develops from this artery or the accompanying vein. In one-third of cases, EDH may be traced to venous sinus bleeding. *(Ref. 1, pp. 426–428; Ref. 2, pp. 366–367)*

7. **T.** Following contusion, early seizures are probably related to hematoma development. Late seizures are probably related to gliosis (scar) formation. Seizures are most likely if any of these features are present:

a. Depressed skull fracture with dural tear
b. Penetrating wound
c. Amnesia lasting longer than 24 hr
d. Seizures developing within 8 weeks after traumatic brain injury. In concussion, risk of seizures is not increased. *(Ref. 2, pp. 362–364)*

8. **T.** These veins enter the dural sinuses and may easily be injured, especially if the brain is atrophic, as in elderly, alcoholic, or Alzheimer's patients. Documented trauma is implicated in only 50% of chronic SDH patients; therefore, the absence of trauma is not helpful in excluding chronic SDH. *(Ref. 1, pp. 428–429)*

9. **T.** The terms "punch drunk" and "dementia pugilistica" are synonymous. Clinical features include extrapyramidal and cerebellar signs, dysarthria, and cognitive impairment. Pathological findings in these patients include substantia nigra degeneration, widespread neurofibrillary tangles, and cerebellar folia scarring. *(Ref. 1, p. 438)*

10. **T.** Skull fracture is referred to as "compound" when there is communication between the scalp laceration and brain parenchyma through depressed bone fragments and lacerated dura. The diagnosis of skull fracture is established by skull radiogram; CT detects evidence of underlying brain contusion but is less sensitive for detecting the actual fracture line. *(Ref. 1, p. 417; Ref. 2, pp. 372–373)*

11. **T.** In some head-injured patients, there is diffuse axonal shearing injury. If the frontal and temporal lobes are injured, this may cause profound neuropsychological disturbances. Neurological deficit may also result from hypoxic-ischemic injury or from effects of sustained intracranial hypertension. *(Ref. 1, pp. 418–419; Ref. 2, p. 364)*

12. **T.** In trauma-induced brain swelling, there is brain edema with increase in extravascular brain water due to impaired blood–brain barrier (vasogenic edema). In addition, there is increase in intravascular brain–blood volume due to cerebral vasodilatation. *(Ref. 1, pp. 418–419)*

13. **F.** Contusions are "bruises." These are usually located in superficial regions such as the undersurfaces of the frontal or temporal lobes. Contusions frequently occur directly beneath skull fracture; however, they may occur in the absence of fracture. They occur at the site of a blow to head (coup injury) or at a site opposite the impact point (contrecoup injury). *(Ref. 1, pp. 419–420; Ref. 2, pp. 362–363)*

14. **F.** EDH are more sharply localized, as they form in *potential* spaces. SDH are more diffuse, crescent-shaped extracerebral lesions and are less well localized. With EDH, look at "scout"

skull radiogram on CT for a fracture line across the middle meningeal artery groove. CT cannot always predict whether a lesion is EDH or SDH; however, *both* types of lesions require surgical intervention if they cause mass effect. *(Ref. 1, pp. 426–428; Ref. 2, pp. 366–367)*

15. **F.** All acute SDH with associated mass effect should be surgically evacuated. Small SDH which do not cause mass effect may *not* require surgery. The patient's clinical condition should be monitored carefully, and serial CT should be performed to determine if SDH size is decreasing or increasing and to determine if mass effect caused by the SDH is increasing or decreasing. Most *small* SDH resolve spontaneously. *(Ref. 1, pp. 428–430)*

16. **T.** An *excessive* accumulation of CSF located in the subdural space is a subdural hygroma. This is caused by trauma. There is tearing of the *arachnoid* and leakage of CSF into the subdural space. Diagnosis is established by CT. Drainage of CSF is usually not needed unless there is large CSF collection. In some cases, shunting of CSF from the subdural hygroma to the subarachnoid space is indicated if the hygroma causes neurological symptoms. *(Ref. 1, p. 431)*

17. **T.** Trauma with carotid artery laceration within the cavernous sinus may cause this fistula. Look for skull radiographic evidence of sphenoid bone fracture. Exam shows orbital bruit due to fistula, exophthalmos, distended orbital veins, cranial nerve (III, IV, VI, V; opthalmic branch) dysfunction. Diagnosis is established by angiogram. *(Ref. 1, p. 433)*

18. **D.** If carotid or vertebral arteries are injured in the neck, dissection of the involved artery with subsequent thrombosis and ischemic stroke may occur. If the carotid artery is injured, sympathetic fibers which travel with this artery may lead to *ipsilateral* Horner syndrome and *contralateral* hemiparesis. Initial symptoms of carotid artery injury may be neck pain or headache. Delayed traumatic brain hemorrhage must be considered but would not be consistent with this clinical pattern, due to the presence of Horner syndrome. With axonal shearing injury, diffuse rather than focal signs would be expected. *(Ref. 1, p. 433)*

19. **C.** Since hemorrhage must always be excluded in traumatic brain injury, CT would be preferable to MRI; however, MRI is more likely to show ischemic brain injury due to carotid artery dissection. LP would be most sensitive to exclude SAH, but this is unlikely with these neurological findings. *(Ref. 2, pp. 261–263)*

20. **E.** If vascular disease is suspected which extends to the *intracranial* region, MRA or a conventional carotid angiogram should be performed. They are more likely to show characteristic angiographic findings of carotid artery wall dissection. Carotid ultrasound would show extracranial carotid artery but would *not* visualize the *intracranial* carotid artery. *(Ref. 2, pp. 56–60)*

21. **A.** The major threat in suspected arterial dissection is that the damaged wall will lead to distal clot propagation, thrombus formation, and carotid occlusion. This could be prevented by anticoagulation. Surgical repair of the damaged (dissected) carotid artery is not indicated. *(Ref. 1, p. 433)*

22. **F.** Stroke is sudden onset of *focal* neurological deficit which rapidly reaches maximal severity. It is unlikely that the patient suffered a vascular event; however, remember to consider carotid artery dissection with this type of injury. The lack of meningeal signs is not consistent with diagnosis of traumatic subarachnoid hemorrhage. *(Ref. 2, pp. 356–370)*

23. **F.** Although it is most likely that the headache is part of the postconcussive syndrome, posttraumatic migraine must be considered although it usually develops at a later time. This diagnosis would be established if the subsequent course was one of recurrent headache episodes. *(Ref. 2, p. 108)*

24. **T.** With persistent (not transient) alteration of consciousness, emergency CT or MRI is warranted to exclude trauma-induced mass lesion. An alternative approach is to have patient observed with serial neurological checks every hour for 24 hr. *(Ref. 2, pp. 361–362)*

25. **F.** Since SAH or meningitis is not considered likely, immediate LP would not be warranted. *(Ref. 2, pp. 54–56)*

26. **A.** Raccoon eyes and Battle sign (indicating blood dissecting along the base of the skull) cranial nerve dysfunction suggest basilar skull fracture. Also, observe for CSF leakage (rhinorrhea, otorrhea). *(Ref. 2, pp. 371–372)*

27. **A.** If basilar skull fracture is suspected, skull radiogram and possibly tomograms are warranted to demonstrate fracture location. The basal skull bones are very thin, and it may be difficult to visualize the fracture radiographically. CT/MRI should be performed to exclude accompanying intracranial injury. *(Ref. 2, pp. 371–372)*

28. **A.** CSF leakage from the nose (rhinorrhea) or ear (otorrhea) is a potential complication. If CSF leakage is demonstrated, perform an isotope cisternogram to demonstrate the location of the fracture and dural tear. This usually occurs with ethmoid or sphenoid bone fracture or orbital plate of frontal bone fracture. In patients with nasal discharge, CSF can be distinguished from nasal secretion because the glucose concentration of CSF is higher than that of nasal secretion. *(Ref. 2, pp. 371–372; Ref. 4, pp. 184–185)*

29. **A.** With dural tear, CSF may become contaminated and bacterial meningitis may occur. This would require LP with CSF exam to establish a diagnosis of meningitis; treatment for 2 weeks with intravenous antibiotics is necessary. *(Ref. 2, pp. 371–372; Ref. 4, pp. 184–185)*

30. **A.** With base of skull fracture, the olfactory nerve is most commonly injured. Patients commonly develop anosmia as a consequence of this traumatic injury. *(Ref. 1, p. 436)*

31. **E.** All listed findings are characteristic of basilar skull fracture. Seizures and focal neurological deficit do not occur unless there is accompanying brain injury. *(Ref. 2, pp. 371–372)*

32. **A.** Following brief loss of consciousness and a short period of amnesia, cerebral concussion is most likely, but serial neurological checks must be done for 24 hr. *(Ref. 2, pp. 361–362)*

33. **A.** Neurological checks for 24 hr are warranted, but no neuroimaging studies appear to be warranted at this time. *(Ref. 2, pp. 361–362; Ref. 4, pp. 178–179)*

34. **B.** A "lucid interval" of 2 hr and then neurological deterioration suggests epidural hematoma. There is a possibility of transtentorial herniation, and with dilated *left* pupil, *left*-sided epidural hematoma would be most likely. *(Ref. 2, pp. 366–367)*

35. **E.** With rapid deterioration, all listed modalities are warranted to control herniation, mass effect, and intracranial hypertension. The sooner surgery is carried out, the better the outcome. *(Ref. 2, pp. 364–365, 366–368)*

17

NEUROLOGICAL MANIFESTATIONS OF SYSTEMIC DISEASE

True or False

1. _____ Seizures are an early manifestation of uremic encephalopathy.

2. _____ The "disequilibrium syndrome" develops within 24 hr after hemodialysis and then resolves spontaneously.

3. _____ "Dialysis dementia" is related to high concentration of calcium and aluminum in the dialysate.

4. _____ Aching, cramping pains which occur on the balls of the feet of diabetic patients and are most intense nocturnally are more likely due to lumbar radiculopathy than to sensorimotor polyneuropathy.

5. _____ Focal neurological deficits may be the presenting manifestation in patients with diabetic ketoacidosis.

6. _____ Alcoholic-induced seizures may occur as long as 1 week after the patient stops drinking.

7. _____ Altered consciousness, eye movement abnormalities, and gait impairment are characteristic features of patients with Korsakoff syndrome.

8. _____ Patients with alcohol-induced seizures should not be treated prophylactically with antiepileptic drugs.

9. _____ The finding of asterixis in the outstretched hands is a characteristic clinical feature of hepatic encephalopathy.

10. _____ Rapid, aggressive correction of hyponatremia with hypertonic saline may lead to development of central pontine myelinolysis.

11. _____ Neurological manifestations of systemic lupus (SLE) erythematous may be due to multiple cerebral infarcts or hemorrhages.

12. _____ Chorea may be the initial neurological manifestation of SLE.

13. _____ Patients with subacute combined system disease may show evidence of myelopathy and neuropathy.

14. _____ Sarcoidosis may cause chronic basilar granulomatous meningitis and hydrocephalus.

Multiple Choice

Choose the most appropriate response.

15. _____ Leukemia may cause which of the following:

A. Intracranial hemorrhage
B. Neoplastic meningitis
C. Cranial nerve palsies
D. Hydrocephalus
E. All of the above

16. _____ Wernicke's encephalopathy includes the following features:

A. Permanent weight loss
B. Ocular palsies
C. Acute confusion
D. B and C
E. A, B, and C

17. _____ Clinical features of neuroleptic malignant syndrome (NMS) include:

A. Fever
B. Rigidity of muscles
C. Rhabdomyolysis
D. Elevated CPK
E. All of the above

18. _____ The most appropriate agent for the treatment of eclamptic seizures is:

A. Ativan
B. Phenytoin
C. Magnesium sulfate
D. Phenobarbital
E. Dexamethasone

19. _____ Hypoparathyroidism may be associated with which of the following:

   A. Altered mentation
   B. Seizures
   C. Pseudotumor cerebri
   D. Chorea
   E. All of the above

20. _____ Hyponatremia may be associated with this disorder:

   A. Status epilepticus
   B. Myopathy
   C. Neuropathy
   D. Dementia
   E. Narcolepsy

21. _____ Hyperthyroidism may be associated with which of the following:

   A. Hearing loss
   B. Myasthenia gravis
   C. Neuropathy
   D. Subarachnoid hemorrhage
   E. Cryptococcal meningitis

Respond based on the clinical history.

J.C. is a 52-year-old man with medically intractable coronary artery disease. He undergoes coronary artery bypass graft. Immediately following surgery, his left hand is weak. Neurological examination shows weakness of grip strength and hand muscle weakness, left eye droopiness and miotic left pupil, and symmetrical reflexes with plantar flexor response. He also has a loud left carotid bruit.

22. _____ The most likely cause of the neurological features is:

   A. Cardiogenic cerebral embolism
   B. Carotid occlusion
   C. Hypoxic-ischemic brain injury
   D. Hemorrhagic cerebral infarction
   E. None of the above

23. _____ The initial diagnostic study should be:

   A. CT
   B. MRI
   C. EEG
   D. EKG
   E. EMG/NCV

24. _____ The most likely explanation of the ocular findings is:

   A. Amaurosis fugax
   B. Midbrain syndrome

   C. Pontine syndrome
   D. Carotid artery injury
   E. Brachial plexus involvement

25. _____ To determine the cause of the carotid bruit, this test should be performed:

   A. Cerebral angiogram
   B. Spiral CT angiogram
   C. MRA
   D. Carotid Doppler duplex ultrasound
   E. No test indicated

26. _____ If carotid stenosis exceeds 60%, consider this treatment:

   A. Coumadin
   B. Aspirin
   C. Ticlopidine
   D. Persantine
   E. Carotid endarterectomy (CEA)

T.P. is a 40-year-old chronic renal failure patient. Following his hemodialysis treatment, he develops myalgias, headache, and muscle twitching. He is witnessed to have a generalized seizure. Following a brief flurry of seizures, he is neurologically normal and all laboratory studies show no significant electrolyte or biochemical abnormalities.

27. _____ What is the most likely etiology of the seizures?

   A. Uremic encephalopathy
   B. Dialysis disequilibrium
   C. Hyponatremia
   D. Subdural hematoma
   E. Cerebral hemorrhage

28. _____ Treatment should include:

   A. Intravenous phenytoin
   B. Intravenous lorazepam
   C. Hypertonic saline
   D. Corticosteroids
   E. Clinical observation

29. _____ Two days later, without further dialysis, he has two more prolonged seizures. Following the seizures, examination shows bilateral plantar extensor responses. Management should include:

   A. EEG and CT
   B. EEG
   C. CT
   D. LP
   E. MRI

30. _____ Complications of maintenance hemodialysis include:

A. Dialysis disequilibrium syndrome
B. Progressive intellectual dysfunction
C. Dialysis dementia
D. Intracranial hemorrhage
E. All of the above

31. _____ Five years later, he develops dysarthria, stuttering, speech apraxia, dementia, and myoclonus. EEG shows marked rhythmical slowing but no periodic discharges. The most probable diagnostic possibility is:

A. Jakob-Creutzfeldt disease (J-C)
B. Binswanger's disease
C. Multiinfarct dementia
D. Chronic meningitis
E. Dialysis encephalopathy

T.R. is a hypertensive man who develops headache and becomes confused. Examination shows right pronator drift, mild confusion, supple neck, hypertensive retinopathy with early papilledema, and BP is 300/200 mmHg.

32. _____ The most likely diagnosis is:

A. Hypertensive encephalopathy (HE)
B. Hypertensive intracerebral hemorrhage
C. Cerebral infarction
D. TIA
E. Subarachnoid hemorrhage (SAH)

33. _____ The initial diagnostic study should be:

A. MRI
B. EKG
C. LP
D. CT
E. Chest radiogram

34. _____ Initial treatment should include:

A. Sublingual procardia
B. Dexamethasone
C. Hyperventilation
D. Mannitol
E. Intravenous nitroprusside

P.R. is a 50-year-old female chronic renal failure patient on chronic hemodialysis who is being prepared for renal transplantation utilizing cyclosporine for immunosuppression. She gradually becomes confused. Examination shows mild inattentional agitated state, intentional tremor, and Anton syndrome. Blood pressure is 220/140 mmHg.

35. _____ Potential etiologies include:

A. Cyclosporine toxicity
B. Hypertensive encephalopathy
C. Uremic encephalopathy
D. Leukoencephalopathy
E. All of the above

36. _____ The most sensitive diagnostic study to establish the cause of this disorder is:

A. EEG
B. LP
C. Noncontrast CT
D. Postconstrast CT
E. MRI

37. _____ Treatment should include:

A. Discontinue or reduce dose of cyclosporine
B. Introduce corticosteroids
C. Utilize calcium channel blockers
D. Both A and C
E. None of the above

38. _____ Neurological manifestations of cyclosporine toxicity include:

A. Tremor
B. Aphasia and apraxia
C. Lymphoma
D. Dementia
E. All of the above

39. _____ This metabolic derangement commonly causes encephalopathy:

A. Hypokalemia
B. Hyperkalemia
C. Hyperglycemia ketoacidosis
D. Hyponatremia
E. All of the above

40. _____ The following is true of hyponatremic encephalopathy:

A. Commonly occurs in alcoholics and malnourished patients
B. Causes central pontine myelinolysis (CPM)
C. CPM occurs unless hyponatremia is rapidly corrected
D. All of the above
E. None of the above

A 22-year-old normotensive woman awakened one night with slurred speech and right-sided weakness. No headache or neck pain was present. She got out of bed and ate breakfast, and symptoms resolved within 30 min. She went back to sleep. When she awakened in the morning, she had slurred speech, right-sided weakness, and sensory disturbance (involving the face, arm, and leg). She had no headache or vomiting.

41. _____ Neurological diagnostic considerations include:

   A. Left middle cerebral artery infarct
   B. Left parietal hemorrhage
   C. Subarachnoid hemorrhage
   D. Left subcortical infarct
   E. Right pontine infarct

42. _____ Important information which may be obtained from the medical history includes:

   A. Prior use of oral contraceptive medication
   B. Family history of stroke
   C. Utilization of over-the-counter cold medications
   D. Use of illicit drugs
   E. All of the above

43. _____ Important diagnostic studies include:

   A. Urine for amino acids
   B. Lactic acid levels
   C. Antiphospholipid antibody determination
   D. Transesophageal echocardiography
   E. All of the above

44. _____ Risk factors for stroke in migraine patients include:

   A. Oral contraceptive pills (OCP)
   B. Hypertension
   C. Cigarette smoking
   D. All of the above
   E. None of the above

J.B. is a 32-year-old woman with systemic lupus erythematous (SLE). She has malar skin rash, arthritis, and renal dysfunction. She is treated with 80 mg of Prednisone daily. She becomes confused and behaves in a psychotic manner with visual hallucinations 48 hr after initiation of corticosteroids.

45. _____ Diagnostic possibilities include:

   A. Steroid psychoses
   B. Lupus-induced CNS vasculitis
   C. Lupus meningoencephalitis
   D. All of the above
   E. None of the above

46. _____ Treatment might include:

   A. Rapid tapering of Prednisone dosage
   B. Increase in Prednisone dosage
   C. Haloperidol
   D. Clozapine
   E. Lithium

47. _____ Common neurological manifestations of SLE include:

   A. Seizures and cognitive impairment
   B. Chorea
   C. Transverse myelitis
   D. Peripheral neuropathy
   E. Polymyositis

Two days following normal spontaneous vaginal delivery, a 28-year-old woman experiences a seizure. She has prolonged confusional state, and examination (12 hr after the seizure) shows isolated right-sided abducens paresis. Blood pressure is 150/95 mmHg.

48. _____ Diagnostic possibilities include:

   A. Venous sinus thrombosis
   B. Hypertensive encephalopathy (HE)
   C. Eclampsia
   D. Subarachnoid hemorrhage (SAH)
   E. Intracerebral hemorrhage

49. _____ The most useful diagnostic study would be:

   A. MR angiogram
   B. Postcontrast CT
   C. LP
   D. MRI
   E. EEG

50. _____ The mechanism of unilateral abducens nerve paresis is:

   A. Cerebral edema
   B. Increased intracranial pressure
   C. Pontine infarct
   D. Cerebral ischemia
   E. None of the above

51. _____ Treatment of this disorder would most likely include:

   A. Corticosteroids
   B. Hyperventilation
   C. Magnesium sulfate
   D. Nitroprusside
   E. Heparin

52. _____ This condition frequently exacerbates during pregnancy:

A. Multiple sclerosis (MS)
B. Migraine
C. Carpal tunnel syndrome
D. Petit mal seizures
E. All of the above

A 48-year-old alcoholic man has been drinking heavily for 2 weeks. He is found confused by his friends, and he becomes increasingly lethargic. He is brought to hospital. Exam shows that he is confused but has no other neurological deficit. He is diaphoretic, tachycardiac, and afebrile.

53. _____ Diagnostic possibilities include:

A. Alcohol-induced encephalopathy
B. Postictal state
C. Hypoglycemia
D. Hepatic encephalopathy
E. All of the above

54. _____ Following treatment with 100 g of glucose intravenously, he remains confused. Examination shows vertical and horizontal nystagmus and gait ataxia. Diagnostic possibilities include:

A. Wernicke syndrome
B. Korsakoff syndrome
C. Hyperglycemia
D. Behavioral status epilepticus
E. None of the above

55. _____ He then develops multiple generalized seizures. Diagnostic possibilities include:

A. Alcohol withdrawal seizures
B. Diabetic ketoacidosis
C. Wernicke syndrome
D. Central pontine myelinolysis
E. Cerebellar degeneration

56. _____ Treatment of seizures should include:

A. Adequate hydration
B. Glucose
C. Thiamine
D. Phenytoin
E. All of the above

57. _____ Two days later, he becomes increasingly confused. Examination shows weakness in both legs and bilateral Babinski signs. Diagnostic possibilities would most likely be:

A. Meningioma
B. Multiple brain abscesses
C. Bilateral subdural hematoma (SDH)
D. Glioblastoma multiforme
E. Multiple metastases

A 38-year-old woman with mitral stenosis and atrial fibrillation suddenly becomes confused. Exam shows agitated inattentive state with left-sided homonymous hemianopsia. The patient is afebrile. Urinalysis shows microscopic hematuria. Complete blood count is normal. She discontinued Coumadin 2 months previously.

58. _____ The most likely diagnosis is:

A. Encephalopathy
B. Postictal state
C. Right middle cerebral artery ischemia
D. Right temporal hematoma
E. None of the above

59. _____ The most likely mechanism of neurological deficit is:

A. Cardiogenic cerebral embolism
B. Thrombotic thrombocytopenic purpura
C. Bacterial endocarditis
D. Hypoxic-ischemic brain injury
E. None of the above

60. _____ The initial diagnostic study which should be performed to determine subsequent management is:

A. Noncontrast CT
B. Blood cultures
C. MRI
D. Transthoracic echocardiogram
E. Transesophageal echocardiogram

61. _____ Management should include:

A. Immediate IV heparin
B. Initiate IV heparin 48 hr later
C. Initiate IV heparin 48 hr later based on CT results
D. Intravenous antibiotics
E. Intravenous antibiotics and heparin

A 43-year-old insulin-dependent diabetic has a left focal motor seizure. Following the seizure, the patient has left hemiparesis-hemianesthesia. CT shows no abnormality. Blood sugar is 780 mg%; blood pH is 7.1; there is no ketonuria; the patient has serum hyperosmolarity.

62. _____ The most likely diagnosis is:

A. Diabetic ketoacidosis
B. Diabetic nonketotic hyperosmolar encephalopathy
C. Diabetic cerebral infarction
D. Uremic encephalopathy
E. None of the above

63. _____ The seizures should be treated with this anticonvulsant:

A. Phenobarbital
B. Phenytoin
C. Carbamazepine
D. Mysoline
E. None of the above

64. _____ Patients with diabetic ketoacidosis almost never develop seizures because of:

A. Hyponatremia
B. Acidosis
C. Ketosis
D. Hyperglycemia
E. Hypokalemia

A 20-year-old obese woman reports new-onset intermittent bifrontal headache. She has developed amenorrhea but no galactorrhea. Exam shows loss of funduscopic venous pulsations, enlarged blind spots, and left lateral rectus paresis.

65. _____ The most likely diagnosis is:

A. Idiopathic intracranial hypertension (IIH)
B. Bifrontal meningioma
C. Pituitary adenoma
D. Empty sella syndrome
E. Craniopharyngioma

66. _____ The most definitive diagnostic study (and the one most likely to establish the diagnosis) is:

A. LP
B. CT
C. MRI with gadolinium contrast
D. Endocrine studies
E. Angiogram

67. _____ LP would most likely show:

A. Elevated opening pressure
B. Acellular fluid
C. Normal protein
D. Normal sugar
E. All of the above

68. _____ Enlargement of the blind spots most commonly indicates:

A. Optic atrophy
B. Retrobulbar neuritis
C. Papilledema
D. Pseudopapilledema
E. None of the above

69. _____ Treatment of this patient should initially include:

A. Acetazolamide
B. Repeat LP with CSF drainage
C. Corticosteroids
D. Optic nerve fenestration
E. All of the above

A 35-year-old man complains of horizontal double vision when reading. He has lost 20 lb over the last 2 months, has insomnia, palpitations, and feels shaky. He has a history of heavy alcohol ingestion and has had prior episodes of delirium tremens. Exam shows bilateral medical rectus paresis, lid lag, slight proptosis, and a pulse rate of 110.

70. _____ The most likely diagnosis is:

A. Wernicke syndrome
B. Myasthenia gravis
C. Myasthenic syndrome
D. Hyperthyroidism
E. Occult neoplasm

71. _____ The most useful diagnostic test would be:

A. Thyroid function studies
B. Tensilon test
C. Chest radiogram
D. EMG/NCV
E. Brain CT with contrast

72. _____ Common causes of extraocular muscle paresis include:

A. Thyroid dysfunction
B. Wernicke syndrome
C. Myasthenia gravis
D. All of the above
E. None of the above

73. _____ Complications of dysthyroid ophthalmopathy include:

A. Visual loss
B. Diplopia
C. Lid lag
D. Loss of accommodation
E. Glaucoma

74. _____ This disorder is commonly associated with hyperthyroidism:

    A. Myasthenia gravis (MG)
    B. Myasthenic syndrome
    C. Bronchogenic carcinoma
    D. Polycythemia
    E. AIDS

75. _____ The following is true of diplopia:

    A. Lateral rectus paresis causes maximal diplopia on far gaze
    B. Medial rectus paresis causes maximal diplopia on far gaze
    C. Lateral rectus paresis causes vertical diplopia
    D. Medical rectus paresis causes head tilt
    E. All of the above

M.M. is an eclamptic woman who develops seizures and is treated with magnesium sulfate. Following this she becomes weak, fatigued, and has double vision. Exam shows proximal muscle weakness and absent deep tendon reflexes.

76. _____ The most likely cause for the neurological symptoms is:

    A. Magnesium sulfate toxicity
    B. Myasthenia gravis (MG)
    C. Myasthenic syndrome
    D. Ascending polyneuropathy
    E. None of the above

77. _____ The most likely location of the neurological abnormality in this condition is:

    A. Spinal cord
    B. Anterior horn cell
    C. Peripheral nerve
    D. Neuromuscular junction
    E. Muscle

78. _____ A serious side effect of magnesium treatment includes:

    A. Encephalopathy
    B. Respiratory arrest
    C. Dysarthria
    D. Absent reflexes
    E. Dysphagia

79. _____ The most effective treatment for eclamptic seizures is:

    A. Magnesium sulfate
    B. Phenytoin

    C. Valproic acid
    D. Phenobarbital
    E. Carbamazepine

80. _____ The most common cause of seizures occurring 1 week postpartum is:

    A. Eclampsia
    B. Hypertensive encephalopathy
    C. Cerebral hemorrhage
    D. Multiple sclerosis
    E. Cortical vein thrombosis

Following surgery for removal of an enlarged and overactive thyroid gland, L.C. noted painful cramping of her fingers and toes. She had abdominal cramps and arching of the back. These cramps were preceded by perioral and acral paresthesias. She had positive Trousseau and Chvostek signs.

81. _____ The patient is describing:

    A. Tetanus
    B. Tetany
    C. Spasticity
    D. Myotonia
    E. None of the above

82. _____ The most common cause of this disorder is:

    A. Hypocalcemia
    B. Hypercalcemia
    C. Hypothyroidism
    D. Hyperthyroidism
    E. None of the above

83. _____ This test could define the nature of this neurological disorder:

    A. Hyperventilation
    B. EMG-NCV
    C. EEG
    D. EKG
    E. Tensilon test

J.B. is a 48-year-old alcoholic with pneumonia, Wernicke syndrome, and hyponatremia. He is treated with multivitamins and rapid correction of hyponatremia utilizing hypertonic fluids. Despite rapid treatment, he becomes weak, lethargic, dysphagic, and has respiratory difficulty.

84. _____ Potential diagnoses include:

    A. Central pontine myelinolysis (CPM)
    B. Basilar artery occlusion
    C. Pontine hemorrhage
    D. All of the above
    E. None of the above

85. _____ Examination would be expected to show:

 A. Quadriplegia
 B. Bilateral Babinski signs
 C. Mutism
 D. Pseudobulbar paresis
 E. All of the above

86. _____ The most useful neurodiagnostic study would be:

 A. EEG
 B. CT
 C. LP
 D. T-1 weighted MRI
 E. T-2 weighted MRI

87. _____ Pathological abnormalities would be expected in this brain region:

 A. Central pons
 B. Subcortical white matter
 C. Basal ganglia
 D. Thalamus
 E. All of the above

88. _____ All but one of the following is characteristic of hyponatremic encephalopathy:

 A. Myopathy
 B. Coma
 C. Status epilepticus
 D. Mutism
 E. Quadriplegia

A 20-year-old man develops chronic diarrhea after eating licorice. He develops weakness and muscle cramps. Exam shows tetany, proximal muscle weakness, and tachypnea.

89. _____ A possible etiology is:

 A. Hyponatremia
 B. Hypercalcemia
 C. Acidosis
 D. Hypokalemia
 E. Hyperglycemia

90. _____ The following finding would not be expected:

 A. Altered mental state
 B. Rhabdomyolysis
 C. Myoglobinuria
 D. Tetany
 E. Myalgias and muscle swelling

91. _____ A potential complication is:

 A. Respiratory arrest
 B. Cardiac arrest
 C. Status epilepticus
 D. Intracerebral hemorrhage
 E. Central pontine myelinolysis

92. _____ The major complication of hyperkalemia may be:

 A. Status epilepticus
 B. Chorea
 C. Cerebral venous sinus thrombosis
 D. Cardiac arrest
 E. Dementia

93. _____ The major complication of hypernatremia is:

 A. Status epilepticus
 B. Intracerebral hemorrhage
 C. Cerebral venous sinus thrombosis
 D. Encephalopathy
 E. All of the above

RESPONSES AND EXPLANATIONS

1. **F.** Seizures are late manifestations unless they are complicating factors such as hyponatremia or hypocalcemia. Also, focal neurological dysfunction is uncommon in renal (metabolic) encephalopathy. Myoclonus and asterixis are common findings. *(Ref. 1, pp. 926–929; Ref. 2, pp. 669–671)*

2. **F.** This includes headache, nausea, cramps, altered mentation, and seizures. This develops immediately or within 24 hr of dialysis. This disorder resolves spontaneously. *(Ref. 1, pp. 926–99; Ref. 2, pp. 669–671; Ref. 4, pp. 286–287)*

3. **F.** This includes speech disturbances including dysarthria, dyspraxia, and mutism; motor disturbances; cognitive impairment; and seizures. EEG shows spike and slow wave patterns. The etiology is *not* known, but high levels of trace elements (aluminum has been especially implicated) in the dialysate may be a causal factor. *(Ref. 1, pp. 928–929; Ref. 2, pp. 669–671; Ref. 4, p. 286)*

4. **F.** In diabetic (and other neuropathies), paresthesias (which may be painful) are worse at night. This is contrasted with intermittent leg claudication due to arterial disease, in which pain increases with exercise and is relieved by rest. Lumbar claudication due to lumbar radiculopathy is exacerbated by prolonged standing. Also, in lumbar radiculopathy, initial sensory symptoms develop over the top rather than the ball (or bottom) of the foot (neuropathy). *(Ref. 2, pp. 671–673)*

5. **F.** In diabetic ketoacidosis, neurological deficit is rarely seen until acidosis becomes severe; however, in nonketotic hyperosmolar states, neurological disturbances (focal neurological deficit or seizures) may be the *initial* manifestation. In all suspected stroke patients, blood sugar should be obtained to exclude this condition. Also, be cognizant that elevated blood sugar may worsen neurological deficit in stroke patients. Remember, ketogenic diet may be used to treat seizures; therefore seizures rarely occur in ketoacidosis. *(Ref. 2, p. 673)*

6. **F.** Alcohol-induced seizures usually occur within 48 hr of cessation of drinking. In alcoholic patients who also have epilepsy, seizures may occur at any time and are precipitated by even small amounts of alcohol. *(Ref. 2, pp. 673–678; Ref. 4, pp. 288–290)*

7. **F.** These findings are characteristic of Wernicke syndrome. This should be treated with thiamine. In Korsakoff syndrome, there is an amnestic syndrome in which patients fail to learn new information and fail to retrieve previously learned facts. Many Korsakoff patients demonstrate confabulation in response to questions for which they cannot respond correctly. *(Ref. 2, pp. 676–677)*

8. **T.** Patients with alcohol-induced seizures develop them because of the direct toxic effect of alcohol. Also, if a patient is taking antiepileptic medication, it is likely that they will suddenly discontinue the medication. This might cause medication-related withdrawal seizures. *(Ref. 2, p. 675; Ref. 4, pp. 288–289)*

9. **F.** Asterixis is seen *most* commonly but not exclusively in hepatic encephalopathy. It may be seen with renal and pulmonary encephalopathy as well as with certain drug intoxications. *(Ref. 1, pp. 915–917; Ref. 2, pp. 678–679)*

10. **T.** CPM may develop due to rapid correction of hyponatremia with hypertonic saline. *(Ref. 2, pp. 677–678)*

11. **T.** Pathological findings in SLE may be varied, including infarcts and hemorrhage possibly due to "vasculitis" or immune-complex formation; however, the exact mechanism of CNS symptoms is not clearly established. Despite pathological evidence of vasculitis, it is *unusual* for an angiogram to show this finding. *(Ref. 1, pp. 952–961; Ref. 2, p. 504)*

12. **T.** Neurological disorders usually occur late in SLE and correlate with severity of renal involvement. Common symptoms include neuropsychiatric disturbances, seizures, and stroke. Less common findings are chorea, transverse myelitis, papilledema, and cranial neuropathies. *(Ref. 1, pp. 952–961; Ref. 2, p. 504)*

13. **T.** In patients with B_{12} deficiency, hematological disturbances including megaloblastic anemia occur. Neurological disturbances may occur even if the patient is not anemic and has no abnormal megaloblasts in blood smear but has a low serum B_{12} level. Clinical manifestations include sensory ataxia, impaired proprioception and vibration sensation, areflexia, and Babinski signs. Rarely, dementia, psychoses, or optic atrophy may result from B_{12} deficiency. *(Ref. 2, pp. 691–692)*

14. **T.** Sarcoid usually causes pulmonary manifestations, and lung biopsy shows noncaesating granulomas. When sarcoid affects the CNS, chronic granulomatous meningitis may occur, causing cranial neuropathies, optic chiasmal, or hypothalamic-pituitary dysfunction. Meningeal (cisternal) involvement may lead to hydrocephalus. *(Ref. 2, pp. 701–702; Ref. 4, pp. 298–299)*

15. **E.** Leukemia can cause coagulation disorders leading to subarachnoid or intracerebral hemorrhage. In addition, if leukemic cells seed into the subarachnoid space, this may cause meningitis. If leukemic cells infiltrate the cranial nerves and basal cisternal spaces, cranial neuropathies and hydrocephalus develop. *(Ref. 1, pp. 906–908)*

16. **D.** Wernicke encephalopathy includes these clinical features:
    a. Altered mental state
    b. Gait ataxia
    c. Eye movement abnormalities
    This disorder most commonly occurs in alcoholic patients and is due to thiamine deficiency. It may also occur in pregnant patients with persistent vomiting. *(Ref. 1, pp. 971–972)*

17. **E.** NMS is precipitated by dopamine-blocking agents (high-potency antipsychotic medication). Because of intense muscle rigidity, elevated CPK and muscle breakdown (rhabdomyolysis) occur. The latter disorder may lead to acute renal failure. Treatment of NMS includes:
    a. Discontinuation of neuroleptic drug
    b. Hydration
    c. Reduce hyperthermia
    d. Bromocriptine (dopamine agonist)
    e. Dantrolene
    (Ref. 2, pp. 519, 649)

18. **C.** Eclampsia is hypertensive disease of pregnancy. Seizures usually respond to lowering of blood pressure. Recent studies indicate that magnesium sulfate is the most effective agent for eclamptic seizures despite the fact that this medication is *not* an effective antiepileptic agent. The component of *vasospasm* in eclampsia has not been established; however, magnesium may act as a vasodilating agent. *(Ref. 1, pp. 962–966; Ref. 2, pp. 705–706)*

19. **E.** In hypoparathyroidism, there is hypocalcemia. This results in central and peripheral nervous system hyperexcitability. With *acute* hypocalcemia, neurological features include mental change, seizures, twitching of the face with palpation over the facial nerve (Chvostek sign), and carpopedal spasm. With chronic hypocalcemia, neurological manifestations include papilledema, cataracts, parkinsonism, mental retardation, and basal ganglia calcification (seen on CT scan). *(Ref. 1, pp. 894–895)*

20. **A.** Hyponatremia results in decreased plasma osmolality and cerebral edema. Clinical features include mental confusion and seizures, including status epilepticus. The risk of neurological disturbances is related to the rapidity of reduction of serum sodium rather than the level of hyponatremia. For example, some patients with a syndrome of inappropriate antidiuretic hormone secretion (e.g., due to pulmonary neoplasm) may be neurologically asymptomatic even with serum sodium of 85 mEq/L because reduction occurred insidiously over several months. *(Ref. 2, pp. 679–681)*

21. **B.** Patients with *hyperthyroidism* may develop:
    a. Adrenergic hyperactivity—tremor, anxiety, insomnia, tachycardia
    b. Ophthalmoplegia with exophthalmos
    c. Myopathy
    d. Myasthenia gravis

Hearing loss is suggestive of *hypothyroidism,* which may also cause ataxia, psychoses, and mental retardation. *(Ref. 1, pp. 892–894)*

22. **E.** Stroke must be considered following any type of cardiovascular procedure; however, weakness which appears confined to the ulnar nerve or the lower portion of the brachial plexus suggests occurrence of a stretch injury. This might result from improper positioning during surgery. The lack of reflex changes and the lack of motor involvement in the face and leg, as well as the normal strength in the remainder of the arm, is not consistent with stroke. Lower brachial plexus lesions (C-8 to T-1) may be due to traction on the abducted arm or compression from a neoplasm of the lung apex (Pancoast syndrome). Horner syndrome, with ptosis and miosis but no anhidrosis, may occur with lower brachial plexus injury. *(Ref. 1, pp. 918–919)*

23. **E.** If hemorrhagic stroke is suspected, CT should be the initial study; and if nonhemorrhagic stroke is suspected, MRI should be the initial diagnostic study. Because stretch injury to the brachial plexus is suspected, EMG-NCV should be the initial study. *(Ref. 1, pp. 918–919)*

24. **E.** With involvement of the undivided anterior primary ramus of T-1, Horner syndrome with miosis and ptosis may be present. Unless preganglionic fibers which travel along the carotid artery are involved, there is no anhidrosis. Amaurosis fugax refers to "fleeting blindness" and is characteristic of transient ischemic attack involving the carotid artery. With carotid TIA, there is ipsilateral blindness (due to retinal ischemia) with contralateral motor and sensory deficit. *(Ref. 1, pp. 918–919; Ref. 2, pp. 717–718)*

25. **D.** This patient with coronary artery disease also most likely has atherosclerotic *cerebrovascular* disease. This may lead to carotid stenosis. The turbulence in the carotid artery causes the bruit. The bruit does *not necessarily* indicate carotid *stenosis.* Bruit may indicate turbulent flow due to abnormal hemodynamics in arterial or venous circulation. Doppler duplex ultrasound study is the best *noninvasive* study to detect extracranial carotid stenosis. Transcranial Doppler shows *intracranial* vessel stenosis. Both spiral CT angiogram and conventional angiogram are *invasive* in that they require *contrast* administration. Since MRA is noninvasive, it is the preferred study after carotid Doppler duplex ultrasound. *(Ref. 2, pp. 255–257)*

26. **E.** Based on recent studies, CEA is indicated in asymptomatic patients with greater than 60% carotid stenosis. Treatment with antiplatelet or anticoagulant medication is not warranted, but cholesterol-lowering agents may reduce stroke risk. *(Ref. 2, pp. 255–257)*

27. **B.** Symptoms are consistent with dialysis "disequilibrium" syndrome. This is due to rapid fluid and electrolyte shifts. Since the patient is neurologically normal following the

seizure, it is unlikely that there is an underlying structural brain lesion. Remember, many chronic dialysis patients are immunosuppressed and have coagulation disturbances; therefore they are at risk for intracranial infectious-inflammatory or hemorrhagic brain lesions. Be careful before concluding that symptoms are related *only* to dialysis disequilibrium. *(Ref. 2, pp. 669–670)*

28. **E.** Because this is usually a self-limited condition, treatment is *not* warranted. If a flurry or burst of prolonged seizures occurs, treatment with intravenous medication (lorazepam, diazepam, phenytoin) would be warranted. If hyponatremia caused the seizure, hypertonic saline is warranted to control seizures. *(Ref. 1, pp. 926–929; Ref. 2, pp. 669–670)*

29. **A.** When seizures persist beyond 24 hr postdialysis, other etiologies must be considered. EEG should be performed to exclude persistent "electrical" status epilepticus, which would require treatment with intravenous antiepileptic medication. Noncontrast CT should be performed to exclude intracranial hemorrhage (intracerebral or subdural). This may develop in chronic renal failure patients due to coagulation disorders and fluid shifts which may occur during dialysis. *(Ref. 2, pp. 670–671)*

30. **E.** All listed features are complications of hemodialysis. The most severe form of progressive intellectual deterioration is "dialysis dementia." The etiology has not been clearly delineated but may be related to the presence of trace elements, e.g., aluminum, within the dialysate. All potential etiologies of dementia must be excluded by appropriate diagnostic studies, e.g., lymphoma, chronic meningitis, subdural hematoma. *(Ref. 2, pp. 670–671)*

31. **E.** The characteristics listed are most consistent with dialysis dementia. Due to prominent EEG abnormalities, use of antiepileptic drugs has been tried, but without success. J-C disease may also be associated with myoclonus, but *periodic* EEG discharges would be expected. In Binswanger's disease and multiinfarct dementia, there is history of multiple prior strokelike episodes. *(Ref. 2, pp. 670–671)*

32. **A.** Acute hypertensive vascular crisis (HE) is characterized by:
    a. Acute marked elevation of blood pressure
    b. Alteration of generalized neurological function (impaired consciousness, generalized seizure), usually with *minimal* focal neurological dysfunction
    c. Funduscopic abnormalities of retinopathy
    In other stroke syndromes, *focal* neurological deficit is prominent with impaired consciousness unless there is marked mass effect or brainstem dysfunction. In SAH, the patient usually has a stiff neck. *(Ref. 4, pp. 154–155)*

33. **D.** CT should be performed to be certain that acute blood pressure elevation has not caused cerebral hemorrhage or in-

farction. CT is usually *normal* in *uncomplicated* HE. *(Ref. 4, pp. 154–155)*

34. **E.** In HE, blood pressure should be lowered carefully, using an agent which can be monitored, titrated, and controlled. Consider labetalol or nitroprusside. Avoid calcium channel blockers or apresoline. The goal is to avoid lowering BP below the cerebral perfusion pressure, as this may result in cerebral ischemia. This perfusion pressure may be higher in chronic hypertensives than in normotensive patients. *(Ref. 4, pp. 154–155)*

35. **E.** Cyclosporine causes CNS neurotoxicity which usually correlates with serum level. It is reversible when the dose is reduced or cyclosporine is discontinued. Reversible white-matter lesions in the parietal-occipital region may develop, consistent with leukoencephalopathy. With marked elevation of BP related to cyclosporine, this disorder could be HE. Because patient has chronic renal failure, uremic encephalopathy may develop in this clinical setting. *(Ref. 1, p. 985)*

36. **E.** MRI is the most sensitive study to establish the diagnosis of white-matter leukoencephalopathy. The gradual development of symptoms is not consistent with intracranial hemorrhage; therefore MRI probably should be performed prior to CT. *(Ref. 1, p. 985)*

37. **A.** Cyclosporine neurotoxicity usually correlates with serum level. Toxicity develops at levels of 500 mg/mL. This disorder (including white-matter lesions) is reversible with reduction of dose. Remember, cyclosporine is a potent hepatic cytochrome P-450 inducer, and this may enhance metabolism of antiepileptic medication. Monitor AED levels carefully in seizure patients receiving cyclosporine. *(Ref. 1, p. 985)*

38. **A.** Clinical features of cyclosporine toxicity include altered consciousness, tremor, seizures, ataxia, and occipital blindness. These are signs of white-matter involvement which are most prominent. Aphasia, apraxia, and dementia indicate gray-matter involvement and occur less commonly. *(Ref. 1, p. 985)*

39. **D.** Abnormalities of potassium metabolism cause muscle weakness. Unless metabolic derangements associated with diabetic acidosis are severe, e.g., lactic acidosis, encephalopathy does not occur. Sodium abnormalities are associated with prominent CNS disturbances, e.g., altered consciousness, seizures. *(Ref. 2, p. 683)*

40. **D.** Hyponatremic encephalopathy which is rapidly corrected may lead to CPM with destruction of white-matter myelin sheaths, especially those located in the basis pontis. Predisposing factors for CPM include alcoholism and chronic malnutrition. MRI is more sensitive than CT for detecting brainstem lesions. Patients with CPM usually deteriorate rapidly and die. *(Ref. 2, pp. 679–681)*

41. **D.** With left-sided (dominant) cerebral hemispheric dysfunction, it is important to differentiate cortical from subcortical involvement. With *cortical* involvement, aphasia and a motor-sensory pattern in which the face and arm are involved to a greater extent than the leg can be expected. With no language dysfunction (dysarthria and not aphasia) and equal involvement of the face, arm, and leg, this is consistent with a subcortical lesion. Lack of headache and vomiting is more consistent with infarct than with hemorrhage. *(Ref. 4, pp. 4–5, 8–11)*

42. **E.** In young patients with stroke, consider nonarteriosclerotic or nonhypertensive etiologies. Illicit drugs including cocaine and amphetamines should be considered strong etiological possibilities to cause stroke. Certain sympathomimetic medications including those contained in appetite suppressants and over-the-counter cold medications may cause stroke. Family history is also a major stroke risk factor. *(Ref. 2, p. 281)*

43. **E.** In young patients with stroke, consider a cardiogenic source, coagulation disorders, and vasculitis. Metabolic disorders including homocystinuria (cystathionine synthetase deficiency) may be associated with arterial and venous thrombosis. There is elevated *urinary* homocystine in patients with homocystinuria. Mitochondrial encephalopathy causing strokelike disorders and seizures shows elevated blood *lactic acid;* ragged-red fibers are seen on muscle biopsy. This condition is due to mitochondrial DNA mutations. *(Ref. 1, pp. 264–271; Ref. 2, p. 281)*

44. **D.** In migraine patients who utilize OCP, there is increased stroke incidence. This correlates with the estrogen content of OCP. Stroke risk in migraine patients is increased by hypertension, cigarette smoking, and family history of stroke. *(Ref. 2, p. 696)*

45. **D.** In patients with SLE, cerebral lupus encephalopathy may develop. These symptoms may be due to small vessel thrombosis with microinfarcts or deposition of brain immune complexes. Symptoms include cognitive impairment, behavioral disturbances, and confusional states. Treatment includes high-dose intravenous methylprednisolone followed by oral prednisone. Unfortunately, side effects of corticosteroids may cause psychotic features similar to symptoms of lupus cerebritis. If symptoms develop soon after initiation of corticosteroids, these behavioral symptoms are probably drug-related rather than due to lupus encephalopathy. *(Ref. 2, p. 504)*

46. **A.** Because psychotic symptoms developed after initiation of corticosteroids, this most likely represents medication effect; therefore rapid tapering of prednisone is warranted. Alternative treatment for CNS SLE includes cyclophosphamide. Utilization of antipsychotic or antimania drugs may be necessary in corticosteroid-treated patients but should initially be avoided. If the neuro-behavioral symptoms are related to *lupus,* it will be necessary to increase the prednisone dosage. *(Ref. 2, p. 504)*

47. **A.** In SLE patients, lupus cerebritis may cause encephalopathy (seizures, cognitive impairment). Uncommon CNS manifestations include chorea and transverse myelitis. In SLE, *peripheral* manifestations include focal neuropathy and polyneuropathy, but these are *uncommon. (Ref. 1, pp. 957–959)*

48. **A.** Neurological manifestations of eclampsia *rarely* occur after pregnancy is terminated. HE usually occurs with higher blood pressure than is demonstrated in this patient. Lack of focal neurological signs is not consistent with intracerebral hemorrhage, and lack of headache is not consistent with SAH. The pattern is consistent with venous sinus thrombosis. This occurs during labor or in the early postpartum period. Occlusion of cerebral veins may lead to venous infarction. Symptoms include focal deficit and seizures; occlusion of venous sinus may lead to increased intracranial pressure due to impaired CSF resorption. *(Ref. 2, pp. 705–706; Ref. 4, pp. 152–153)*

49. **A.** MR angiogram is the most sensitive noninvasive study for showing *venous* occlusion directly. CT and MRI may indirectly show evidence of venous occlusion as manifested by brain parenchymal abnormalities or signs that there is a clot in the venous sinus (e.g., empty delta sign) due to venous occlusion (infarction, hemorrhage). *(Ref. 2, pp. 299–300; Ref. 4, pp. 152–153)*

50. **B.** With occlusion of venous sinus, increased intracranial pressure (ICP) occurs. Diplopia due to abducens nerve paresis results from increased ICP. *(Ref. 2, pp. 299–300; Ref. 4, pp. 152–153)*

51. **E.** Use of anticoagulant (heparin) and thrombolytic (urokinase) agents is effective treatment. If there is increased ICP, treatment with acetazolamide may be effective. If there is cerebral edema, consider corticosteroids. *(Neurology Clinics of North America 10, p. 87, 1992; Ref. 2, pp. 299–300; Ref. 3, pp. 152–153)*

52. **C.** MS does not exacerbate during pregnancy but, due to physical and emotional stress which occur in the *postpartum period,* symptoms may worsen then. Migraine usually goes into remission during pregnancy, and medication treatment is infrequently an issue. Seizures usually do not increase or decrease during pregnancy, but AED levels may fluctuate due to changes in protein drug binding and metabolism. Compression focal neuropathies including the median and facial nerves may exacerbate during pregnancy. These neuropathies usually remit after delivery. Surgery or corticosteroids are rarely necessary treatment. *(Ref. 2, pp. 704–707)*

53. **C.** Alcohol may cause acute fatty liver, hepatitis, or cirrhosis. This decreases available glycogen and may lead to hypoglycemia. Neurological manifestations of hypoglycemia are consistent with metabolic encephalopathy, and there may be sympathomimetic features (diaphoresis, tachycardia). The lack of tremor is *not* consistent with acute delirium tremens. *(Ref. 1, pp. 915–917; Ref. 2, pp. 678–679)*

54. A. The clinical features indicate Wernicke encephalopathy. This alcoholic patient is thiamine depleted but did not have clinical features of Wernicke until he received a glucose bolus. This utilized the small remaining amount of thiamine and the patient then became symptomatic from thiamine depletion. Moral: Utilize thiamine with glucose bolus in a suspected alcoholic patient even if *initially* there are no signs of Wernicke encephalopathy. *(Ref. 1, pp. 967–976; Ref. 2, pp. 677–678)*

55. A. Seizures frequently occur after withdrawal from alcohol. Seizures are not part of the other listed conditions. *(Ref. 2, pp. 676–679; Ref. 4, pp. 288–289)*

56. E. For acute seizure management, a loading dose of intravenous phenytoin is warranted; however, if the patient had only a single seizure, phenytoin treatment is not warranted. It is not indicated to give alcoholic patients prophylactic AED, since they will most certainly *rapidly* and *abruptly* discontinue AED when the next alcoholic binge (which lowers the seizure threshold) occurs. *(Ref. 2, pp. 349–350; Ref. 4, pp. 288–289)*

57. C. Alcoholic patients have brain atrophy and coagulation disturbances and are predisposed to trauma. This is an ideal circumstance for SDH to develop. Since findings involve both legs, consider *bilateral SDH*. Bilateral SDH may be difficult to diagnose with CT/MRI because there may be only subtle signs of mass effect. *(Ref. 2, p. 678)*

58. C. Cardiogenic cerebral embolism has occurred in this patient with valvular atrial fibrillation because the patient is *not* presently being anticoagulated. The lack of headache and vomiting is evidence against temporal hematoma. Microscopic hematuria would indicate renal infarction due to renal embolus. The presence of focal deficit is not consistent with encephalopathy alone. *(Ref. 2, pp. 268–270)*

59. A. Cardiogenic cerebral embolism occurs in patients with valvular atrial fibrillation. Patients with valvular disease are at risk for developing bacterial endocarditis, so multiple blood cultures should be performed. In hypoxic-ischemic brain injury, there are usually no focal neurological signs. Diagnosis of TTP is established by these features:
a. Neurological disturbances
b. Thrombocytopenia
c. Hemolytic anemia
d. Fever
e. Renal impairment
Since CBC and platelet count are normal, TTP is not the diagnosis. *(Ref. 2, pp. 281, 695)*

60. A. Noncontrast CT should be done to determine if an ischemic lesion is present. Ascertain whether the ischemic lesion has undergone hemorrhagic transformation, especially if anticoagulation is being considered. Also, *if* bacterial endocarditis

occurred, mycotic aneurysm may be present and may rupture to cause intracerebral or subarachnoid bleeding. Since the patient is afebrile and the white blood cell count is normal, bacterial endocarditis is unlikely. *(Ref. 2, pp. 268–270)*

61. C. Hemorrhagic transformation of ischemic infarct due to cardiogenic cerebral embolism usually occurs within 48 hr of stroke onset. Wait 48 hr and then initiate heparin as long as CT does not show hemorrhagic transformation. This delay avoids potential bleeding complication but leaves the patient unprotected for recurrent embolism during this 48-hr period. *(Ref. 2, pp. 268–270)*

62. B. This disorder may present with focal seizure or strokelike onset. Potential mechanisms for focal neurological deficit include hyperosmolar state, acidosis, hypotension, dehydration, and intravascular coagulation. Neurodiagnostic studies usually show no abnormality. Neurological dysfunction improves following correction of the metabolic abnormality. Neurological disturbances do *not* develop in diabetic ketoacidosis. *(Ref. 2, p. 673)*

63. E. As for seizures due to any underlying metabolic abnormality, correct the metabolic abnormality and it is usually *not* necessary to use an AED unless status epilepticus occurs as a consequence of metabolic derangement. Following correction of the metabolic abnormality, prophylactic AED are *not* necessary. Also, phenytoin has an effect on glucose metabolism. *(Ref. 2, p. 673)*

64. C. As contrasted with *nonketotic* hyperosmolar states, diabetic ketoacidosis is uncommonly associated with seizures or other neurological disturbances. Remember that *ketogenic* diet is utilized for certain seizure disorders and perhaps *ketosis* of the diabetic state is *protective* against seizures. *(Ref. 2, p. 673)*

65. A. IIH (also referred to as benign intracranial hypertension or pseudotumor cerebri) is characterized by symptoms (headache, vomiting, episodic visual blurring, double vision) and signs (papilledema, lateral rectus paresis, decreased visual acuity) of intracranial hypertension. This condition most commonly occurs in obese women with menstrual irregularity. The lack of galactorrhea is inconsistent with prolactin-secreting pituitary neoplasm. *(Ref. 2, pp. 700–701)*

66. A. All diagnostic studies are negative with the exception of lumbar puncture, which shows *only* elevated opening pressure. CT and MRI exclude a mass lesion or hydrocephalus. Angiogram excludes venous sinus occlusion, which may simulate clinical presentation of IIH. *(Ref. 2, pp. 700–701; Ref. 4, pp. 284–485)*

67. E. LP shows an elevated opening pressure. The finding of *acellular* CSF excludes infectious-inflammatory processes. CSF protein may be elevated in conditions in which the blood–

brain barrier is impaired; *however*, in IIH, protein is normal or low due to increased CSF production, which acts to dilute the protein content. *(Ref. 2, pp. 700–701; Ref. 4, pp. 284–285)*

68. **C.** Enlargement of blind spots is most commonly seen in papilledema; however, rarely in congenital optic disk anomalities such as drusen (pseudopapilledema), blind spots may be enlarged. Scotoma are most common with optic or retrobulbar neuritis. *(Ref. 2, pp. 184, 201)*

69. **E.** In most cases of IIH, treatment with acetazolamide (may reduce CSF production) or repeated LP with drainage of large amounts of CSF cause remission. Prednisone may also be effective even though there is *no* cerebral edema. Because the major threat in IIH is compression of the optic nerve, optic nerve fenestration to relieve optic nerve pressure may be necessary. Rarely, lumbar peritoneal diversionary shunt is necessary to lower CSF pressure and reduce headache. *(Ref. 2, pp. 700–701)*

70. **D.** Despite the patient being an alcoholic and having had prior delirium tremens, systemic manifestations and eye movement abnormalities are most consistent with hyperthyroidism, especially the lid lag and proptosis. Fatigue is present, and this is consistent with myasthenia gravis. *(Ref. 2, pp. 684–685)*

71. **A.** Clinical features are so consistent with hyperthyroidism that results of thyroid function tests should precede any other diagnostic studies. *(Ref. 2, pp. 684–65)*

72. **D.** When patients report diplopia and demonstrate extra-ocular muscle paresis, consider all listed choices. Obviously, there are multiple other causes (listed in the references); however, always consider these three conditions initially. *(Ref. 2, pp. 684–685; Ref. 4, pp. 104–105)*

73. **A.** Ocular findings develop in patients after medical or surgical treatment or hyperthyroidism. Dysthyroid ophthalmopathy can worsen such that the eyeball becomes immobile, visual acuity is impaired, and corneal ulceration develops. Corticosteroids or surgical orbital decompression are warranted when vision is threatened. *(Ref. 1, pp. 692–694; Ref. 2, pp. 684–685)*

74. **A.** MG occurs commonly in hyperthyroid patients. Both these conditions may cause muscle weakness, abnormal fatigue, and abnormal eye movements. *(Ref. 1, pp. 692–694)*

75. **A.** With far gaze, the eyes diverge and this involves the lateral recti muscles. Diplopia is therefore maximal with far gaze. With near gaze, the eyes converge and this involves the medial recti muscles. Diplopia due to medial rectus weakness is maximal when reading. Head tilt occurs with superior oblique muscle weakness. *(Ref. 4, pp. 104–105)*

76. **A.** Treatment of eclamptic seizures with magnesium sulfate may lead to symptoms of neuromuscular junction toxicity. The absent reflexes are not consistent with MG; proximal weakness is not consistent with polyneuropathy. *(Archives of Neurology 45, p. 1360, 1988; Ref. 1, pp. 962–966)*

77. **D.** Magnesium sulfate toxicity affects the *neuromuscular junction*. Other such neuromuscular transmission defect disorders include MG, myasthenic syndrome, botulism, and tick paralysis. *(Archives of Neurology 45, p. 1360, 1988)*

78. **B.** Serious complications of magnesium sulfate toxicity include respiratory depression and cardiac arrhythmias. *(Clinical Obstetrics & Gynecology 35, p. 365, 1992)*

79. **A.** Management of eclamptic seizures is controversial. There is no good evidence that magnesium sulfate is an effective anticonvulsant or that it even crosses the blood–brain barrier. Despite this, one recent study showed that it is more effective than phenytoin in eclamptic seizures, possibly due to the role of vasospasm in causing neurological manifestations of eclampsia. *(American Journal of Obstetrics & Gynecology 166, p. 1757, 1992)*

80. **E.** Neurological manifestations of eclampsia do not usually occur in the postpartum period. Venous sinus and cortical vein thrombosis are the most common causes of seizures. *(Ref. 1, pp. 285–289; Ref. 2, pp. 299–230)*

81. **B.** Tetany is characterized by prolonged limb muscle spasm, laryngospasm, and hyperexcitability of peripheral nerves (Trousseau, Chvostek signs). Painful paresthesias may precede spasms. Spasms may lead to abnormal limb posturing, simulating dystonia. In this condition, peripheral nerves are hyperexcitable, with abnormal reaction to limb ischemia (Trousseau sign) and percussion (Chvostek sign). *(Ref. 1, pp. 792–794)*

82. **A.** Tetany most commonly occurs in hypocalcemia, hypomagnesemia, or alkalosis. It may be precipitated by hyperventilation (respiratory alkalosis). Following thyroid surgery, there may be damage to the adjacent parathyroid gland, which may lead to hypocalcemia. *(Ref. 1, pp. 792–794)*

83. **B.** Peripheral nerve hyperexcitability may be demonstrated by the findings of EMG-NCV with rapid independent discharge rates of motor units. *(Ref. 1, pp. 792–794)*

84. **D.** CPM is characterized by destruction of myelin sheaths in the basis pontis. Most patients are malnourished and alcoholics. They have hyponatremia, and CPM develops after rapid correction of hyponatremia. Clinical features could be consistent with brainstem infarction due to basilar artery occlusion or pontine hemorrhage. *(Ref. 1, pp. 828–829)*

85. **E.** Additional features include ophthalmoparesis, hyper-reflexia, seizures, behavioral disorders, and dysarthria. There may be pathological evidence of *extrapontine* myelinolysis, e.g., thalamus, basal ganglia. *(Ref. 1, pp. 828–829)*

86. **E.** Demyelinating disorders are sensitively detected by T-2 weighted MRI. These demyelinated lesions appear white on T-2 weighted images. T-1 weighted MRI is less sensitive, and lesions may appear dark. *(Ref. 1, pp. 828–829)*

87. **A.** In CPM, pathological lesions are expected in the basis pontis; however, they may be seen in the other regions in *extrapontine* myelinolysis. *(Ref. 1, pp. 828–829)*

88. **A.** Hyponatremia causes CNS effects; therefore myopathy and neuropathy are *not* expected findings. *(Ref. 2, pp. 679–681)*

89. **D.** Certain drugs, e.g., diuretics, amphotericin, and licorice (glycyrrhizate), cause hypokalemia. Excessive urinary and gastrointestinal loss may cause hypokalemia. Hypo- and not hypercalcemia causes tetany. Hyponatremia causes seizures and encephalopathy. *Recovery* from diabetic ketoacidosis may result in hypokalemia. *(Ref. 1, pp. 781–783; Ref. 2, p. 683)*

90. **A.** With hyper- and hypokalemia, peripheral nervous system effects occur. The use of oral potassium supplement may prevent hypokalemia. With hyperkalemia, attacks of muscle weakness may be terminated by administration of calcium gluconate, glucose, and insulin. Acetazolamide may reduce the number of attacks of hyperkalemic weakness. *(Ref. 1, pp. 781–783; Ref. 2, p. 683)*

91. **A.** With severe hypokalemia, there may be bulbar weakness and respiratory depression. *(Ref. 1, pp. 781–783; Ref. 2, p. 683)*

92. **D.** The major risk of hyperkalemia is sudden death due to cardiac arrhythmias. *(Ref. 1, pp. 783–784)*

93. **E.** This occurs in infants and elderly patients. It results from water loss. This may result in sodium excess, especially in patients with impaired thirst and reduced fluid intake. There is extracellular hyperosmolarity and intracellular dehydration. Fluid and electrolyte shifts may lead to the listed neurological disturbances. *(Ref. 2, p. 681)*

18

IMPAIRED CONSCIOUSNESS— STUPOR AND COMA

True or False

1. _____ Central neurogenic hyperventilation may result from midbrain lesions.

2. _____ Decorticate posturing results from a cerebral hemispheric lesion.

3. _____ Decerebrate posturing results from midbrain and upper pontine lesions.

4. _____ In metabolic-induced coma, pupils are invariably normal unless the coma is due to medications which directly affect pupillary size and reactivity.

5. _____ In pontine hemorrhage, pupils are miotic and nonreactive.

6. _____ Ocular bobbing is seen in a comatose patient with bilateral cerebral hemispheric lesions.

7. _____ The finding of absent oculocephalic reflex suggests that the brainstem is not functioning normally.

Multiple Choice

Respond based on the clinical history.

Jack Daniels is a 52-year-old alcoholic man with cirrhosis. After drinking excessively, he becomes confused after falling in a bar and hitting his head. He is brought to the hospital by his friends. On examination, he is disoriented with asterixis and appears icteric; the remainder of the neurological exam is normal.

8. _____ Based on the clinical data, the most useful initial diagnostic study is:

   A. EEG
   B. CT
   C. LP
   D. MRI
   E. Arterial blood ammonia level

9. _____ The most likely diagnosis is:

   A. Bilateral subdural hematoma (SDH)
   B. Unilateral subdural hematoma
   C. Subarachnoid hemorrhage (SAH)
   D. Midbrain hemorrhage
   E. Hepatic encephalopathy

10. _____ With adequate hydration, Jack becomes alert, but 2 days later he deteriorates and becomes confused, develops horizontal and vertical nystagmus, and cannot walk due to gait ataxia. Diagnostic possibilities include:

    A. Central pontine myelinolysis
    B. Wernicke encephalopathy
    C. Hyponatremia
    D. All of the above
    E. None of the above

11. _____ He improves with treatment but again worsens 2 days later. He is now obtunded with bilateral plantar extensor signs. The initial diagnostic study should be:

    A. EEG
    B. LP
    C. CT
    D. MRI
    E. Blood ammonia level

12. _____ Diagnostic considerations include:

    A. Central pontine myelinolysis (CPM)
    B. Brain abscess
    C. Bilateral subdural hematoma
    D. Subarachnoid hemorrhage
    E. All of the above

P.T. is a hypertensive man who falls from a Mardi Gras float. He was conscious on arrival at the Emergency Department, but now (60 min) he is unresponsive. Neurological findings are: pupils, right 2 mm, left 5 mm, both sluggishly reactive; eye movements, none to command; vestibulo-ocular ("Doll's head") are positive;

respirations, tachypneic and spontaneous; motor response, nail-bed pressure to right thumb causes poorly localizing movements of that extremity and bending of right knee, nailbed pressure to left thumb causes flexion at the elbow and extension of the left knee; reflexes, left positive Babinski sign.

13. _____ What is the most likely diagnosis?

    A. Right pontine hemorrhage
    B. Right cerebellar hemorrhage
    C. Right intraventricular hemorrhage
    D. Right frontal subdural hemorrhage
    E. Right midbrain ischemic stroke

Uncle Herniation, Aunt Fossa, and their nephew, Peter Falx (an intern at Charity Hospital), go to Bourbon Street. After two Hurricanes (strong alcoholic drinks), Aunt Fossa complains of severe dizziness and falls to the floor. Her pupils are pinpoint but appear not to respond to iced vodka and tonic squirted in each ear (the local version of the iced water caloric test). Her breathing is gasping at times, then trails off. Sometimes she extends all extremities in decerebrate posture.

14. _____ Aunt Fossa has suffered from:

    A. Hurricane intoxication
    B. Thalamic ischemic stroke
    C. Cerebellar hemorrhage
    D. Pontine hemorrhage
    E. Lateral medullary ischemic stroke

The EMT take Aunt Fossa to the nearest hospital, and Peter looks around for Uncle Herniation. He finds him slumped in a corner drooling out of the left side of his mouth. His breathing is regular but shallow; his pupils are midrange and reactive but his eyes deviate downward; iced vodka and tonic squirted into both ears causes deviation of eyes toward stimulus with some nystagmus. This is accompanied by a generous gush of liquid from the mouth. His left arm and leg are flaccid.

15. _____ Peter Falx is now concerned about ever going to Bourbon Street with Aunt and Uncle again because Uncle Herniation may have suffered:

    A. Hurricane intoxication
    B. Right thalamic ischemic stroke
    C. Cerebellar hemorrhage
    D. Pontine hemorrhage
    E. Lateral medullary ischemic stroke

Matching

Match the clinical features with the pathological condition.

    A. Ataxia, bradycardia, respiratory slowing, elevated blood pressure
    B. Coma, quadriplegia, miotic but reactive pupils, absent Doll's eye
    C. Coma, dilated left pupil, right hemiplegia
    D. Confusion, dilated left pupil, right homonymous hemi-anopsia, aphasia
    E. Confusion, negative Babinski signs, asterixis, normal motor function

16. _____ Metabolic encephalopathy

17. _____ Cerebellar hemorrhage

18. _____ Pontine hemorrhage

19. _____ Left temporal lobe glioblastoma

20. _____ Left subdural hematoma

Match the clinical features with the diagnosis.

    A. Lethargy, appears alert but not responsive, spontaneous eye movements, mute but not paralyzed
    B. Eyes open, may make sound, does not speak or respond, responds to threat, may have reflex movements
    C. Immobile, unable to move limbs, can not speak but moves eyes
    D. Appears akinetic and mute, normal neurological examination, limbs rigid
    E. No spontaneous respiration, no response to pain, coma, negative caloric test, fixed dilated pupils

21. _____ Brain death

22. _____ Catatonia

23. _____ Akinetic mutism

24. _____ Locked-in syndrome

25. _____ Chronic vegetative state (CVS)

RESPONSES AND EXPLANATIONS

1. **T.** Respiratory patterns may have localizing value in comatose patients. High-amplitude rapid respirations may be seen in metabolic acidosis and hypoxia but may also occur with midbrain disease, such as large brainstem hematomas. Irregular respiratory patterns (apneustic, cluster) indicate serious brainstem disease. Cheyne-Stokes respiration indicates bilateral cerebral hemispheric disease. The accompanying neurological disturbances are also important in localizing the lesion. *(Ref. 1, pp. 20–22; Ref. 2, pp. 229–230)*

2. **T.** This is a reflex motor response in which the arms are adducted and flexed and the legs extend. It is caused by cerebral hemispheric lesion. *(Ref. 1, p. 20; Ref. 2, p. 233)*

3. **T.** This is a reflex motor response in which the patient extends, adducts, and internally rotates the arms and extends the legs. It is indicative of bilateral corticospinal and corticobulbar lesion at the midbrain or pontine level. *(Ref. 2, p. 233)*

4. **T.** In comatose patients, normal (midrange and reactive) pupils are most consistent with toxic-metabolic encephalopathy. Usually, there will also be symmetrical motor response and symmetrical oculocephalic and oculovestibular responses. *(Ref. 2, p. 234)*

5. **F.** In pontine hemorrhage, the pupils are miotic and reactive due to bilateral sympathetic dysfunction (the pathway travels in the lateral portion of the brainstem). There is sparing of the parasympathetic fibers of the oculomotor nerve which emerge at midbrain level and are unaffected in pontine hemorrhage. Light reactivity is preserved because the afferent (sensory) portion of the light reflex and the efferent parasympathetic component are preserved. *(Ref. 2, p. 234; Ref. 4, pp. 34–35)*

6. **F.** Rapid downgaze succeeded by slow upgaze occurs in comatose patients with *pontine* lesions. Ocular bobbing occurs because there is impaired *horizontal* eye movement. *(Ref. 2, pp. 235–236)*

7. **T.** The oculocephalic (Doll's head) reflex suggests that the brainstem is not functioning. If it is absent, the oculovestibular (caloric) reflex must then be performed utilizing cold water. Be aware that overdosage with CNS depressant and psychotropic medication may cause caloric reflex to be *transiently* absent. *(Ref. 1, pp. 20–22; Ref. 2. pp. 236–237)*

8. **E.** Although "confusion" occurred after the fall, nonfocal neurological exam with presence of asterixis (which is most consistent with metabolic encephalopathy) in an icteric (jaundiced) patient suggests hepatic encephalopathy. In this case, *arterial* (not venous) blood ammonia level will be elevated. If it is elevated, this *does not exclude* traumatic hematoma, as this lesion frequently occurs in patients with liver disease who have impaired coagulation factors. If traumatic hematoma was present, focal neurological findings would be expected. Be careful not to miss an *accompanying* intracerebral hemorrhage in this patient with hepatic encephalopathy; CT should be performed. *(Ref. 2, p. 678)*

9. **E.** This pattern suggests *metabolic* encephalopathy due to hepatic dysfunction. *Bilateral* SDH would cause bilateral motor deficit (pronator drift, Babinski signs), but since they are absent, this diagnosis is unlikely. *(Ref. 2, p. 239)*

10. **D.** As hydration is improved, fluids without saline, e.g., dextrose and water, may cause hyponatremia. The most serious neurological complication of hyponatremia is *seizures*. Central pontine myelinolysis is characterized by quadriplegia, mutism, and eye movement abnormalities. If an alcoholic patient is given glucose-containing fluids without thiamine supplementation, this may induce Wernicke syndrome (gait dysfunction, confusion, eye movement abnormalities). *(Ref. 2, pp. 679–681)*

11. **C or D.** Alcoholic patients frequently show cerebral atrophy. With adequate treatment and fluid shifts, consider SDH and perform CT or MRI. Focal structural supratentorial (not infratentorial) lesion is suspected based on bilateral Babinski signs without brainstem signs. *(Ref. 2, p. 678)*

12. **C.** Bilateral SDH is most likely. There is no hint of infection to suggest brain abscess. Lack of brainstem signs is not consistent with CPM. *(Ref. 2, pp. 23?–241)*

13. **D.** In a patient who suffered head trauma, SDH is most likely even though the patient is hypertensive. With significant mass effect, transtentorial herniation occurs with compression of the ipsilateral oculomotor nerve and corticospinal tract of the midbrain region. This would cause *ipsilateral* pupillary dilatation and *contralateral* hemiparesis. In unusual cases, herniation causes the upper midbrain to be pushed to the contralateral side so that the dilated pupil is contralateral to the mass lesion. *(Ref. 2, pp. 239–240, 367–369)*

14. **D.** In pontine hemorrhage the following are seen:
    a. Coma
    b. Quadriplegia and decerebration
    c. Absent eye movements (including ocular bobbing)
    d. Miotic but reactive pupils
    e. Abnormal respiratory pattern
    (Ref. 2, pp. 240, 289)

15. **B.** In thalamic hemorrhage, there is contralateral *hemiplegia-anesthesia* with downward ocular deviation with paralysis of upward gaze. Due to intact brainstem, oculovestibular response is intact. *(Ref. 2, p. 288)*

16. **E**
17. **A**
18. **B**
19. **D**
20. **C**

16–20. In metabolic encephalopathy, there are usually no *focal* neurological signs; myoclonus and asterixis are common features. In cerebellar hemorrhage, there may be Cushing reflex (hypertension, bradycardia, respiratory slowing) plus ataxia. For pontine hemorrhage, findings are outlined in Question 14. With left intraaxial (intracerebral) neoplasm, aphasia and visual field defect are characteristic; whereas with extraaxial SDH, there is evidence of transtentorial herniation (ipsilateral pupillary dilatation and contralateral hemiplegia. *(Ref. 2, pp. 240, 288–289)*

21. **E**
22. **D**
23. **A**
24. **C**
25. **B**

21–25. In *brain death*, there is no motor response, pupils are fixed and dilated, and brainstem reflexes are absent. In *catatonia*, the patient appears akinetic and mute, but neurological exam is otherwise normal. With movement of limbs, waxy flexibility may occur as limbs remain in the same position in which they were initially placed. In *akinetic mutism*, the patient appears alert but is not responsive and may have spontaneous eye movements. There is minimal motor response or speech, but the patient is not paralyzed. This is usually caused by a basal bifrontal lesion. In *locked-in syndrome* due to ventral pontine lesion, the patient is quadriplegic with bulbar paralysis but preserved eye movements. Since the dorsal pons is intact with sparing of the ascending reticular activating system (ARAS), the patient is alert. In *CVS*, the patient has severe injury to the bilateral cerebral cortices and subcortical region but the brainstem is relatively spared. This is usually due to severe diffuse hypoxic-ischemic brain injury. The patient appears awake with eyes open but responds only to reflex activities. The patient does not speak or respond to verbal commands. Reflex motor responses (decerebration, decortication) may occur. Cardiovascular and respiratory function are normal. EEG may show some normal alpha activity, and sleep pattern is maintained. *(Ref. 2, pp. 239–242; Ref. 4, pp. 36–37)*

19

DEMYELINATING DISORDERS

True or False

1. _____ The diagnosis of clinically probable multiple sclerosis (MS) is based upon dissemination of symptoms and signs in a temporal and spatial pattern.

2. _____ A major disabling feature in MS patients is fatigue.

3. _____ Lhermitte sign is pathognomonic of MS.

4. _____ Seizures and cognitive decline are common clinical features of MS.

5. _____ Patients with MS are frequently heat sensitive such that neurological deficit worsens in a warm environment.

6. _____ The presence of gadolinium-enhancing MRI lesions is indicative of active MS exacerbation.

7. _____ Caucasian patients of Northern European extraction are more susceptible to MS than are Asian and African patients.

8. _____ The immune-mediated attack in MS is probably directed toward the oligodendrocytes in the CNS.

9. _____ Amantadine (Symmetrel) is effective in treating fatigue in MS patients.

10. _____ Trigeminal neuralgia may be the initial and sole presenting feature of MS.

11. _____ The characteristic pathological lesion in MS is loss of myelin with relative preservation of axons and loss of myelin-producing oligodendrocytes.

12. _____ In patients with optic neuritis, high-dose corticosteroids (intravenous methylprednisolone) has been shown to delay the onset of MS.

Matching

Match the clinical feature with the appropriate statement.

A. Bilateral internuclear ophthalmoplegia (INO)
B. Neuromyelitis optica
C. Charcot triad
D. Transverse myelitis
E. Visual hallucinations

13. _____ Devic disease

14. _____ Symptom of progressive multifocal leukoencephalopathy (PML)

15. _____ Thoracic spinal cord demyelination

16. _____ Characteristic brainstem finding of MS

17. _____ Brainstem and cerebellar demyelination

Multiple Choice

Choose the most appropriate response.

18. _____ Characteristic clinical course(s) of MS are:

A. Exacerbating-remitting
B. Chronic progressive
C. Relapsing-progressive
D. Asymptomatic
E. All of the above

19. _____ Elevated CSF gamma-globulin content may be seen in which of these conditions?

A. MS
B. SLE
C. Neurosyphilis
D. Sarcoid
E. All of the above

20. _____ Interferon has been demonstrated to be effective in this pattern of MS:

A. Exacerbating-remitting
B. Exacerbating-chronic progressive
C. Chronic progressive
D. Optic neuritis
E. Transverse myelitis

21. _____ As a diagnostic test for multiple sclerosis, MRI is:

    A. Highly sensitive and highly specific
    B. Highly sensitive but poorly specific
    C. Poorly sensitive but highly specific
    D. Poorly sensitive and poorly specific
    E. None of the above

Respond based on the clinical history.

Eight days following a viral illness, M.S. develops numbness in his feet, difficulty walking, and bladder incontinence. Examination shows flaccid paraparesis, absent knee, ankle, and abdominal reflexes, bilateral Babinski signs, and sensory level at T-6.

22. _____ The most likely diagnosis is:

    A. Spinal cord metastases
    B. Epidural abscess
    C. Multiple sclerosis
    D. Acute transverse myelopathy
    E. Devic disease

23. _____ Diagnostic studies should include:

    A. Myelogram
    B. Lumbar puncture
    C. Spinal MRI
    D. All of the above
    E. None of the above

24. _____ CSF findings which would confirm the diagnosis of MS include:

    A. Lymphocytosis
    B. Elevated protein content
    C. Oligoclonal bands
    D. Elevated gamma-globulin content
    E. None of the above

25. _____ Treatment should be initiated with:

    A. High-dose intravenous corticosteroids
    B. Plasmapheresis
    C. Interferon
    D. Cytoxan
    E. All of the above

26. _____ The finding of three periventricular high-signal-intensity lesions on T-2 weighted brain MRI suggests this diagnosis:

    A. SLE
    B. Sarcoidosis
    C. Neurosyphilis
    D. Multiple sclerosis
    E. All of the above

H.M. is a 26-year-old paralegal who suffers flexion-extension injury to her neck in a motor vehicle accident. Exam shows loss of cervical lordosis and muscle spasm. Neck pain and stiffness resolve within 4 days following treatment with physical therapy and medication. One week later she complains of numb feet, difficulty walking, and blurred vision in her right eye. Exam shows paraparesis, bilateral Babinski signs, positive Lhermitte sign, loss of proprioception, pinprick and vibration to C-6 level, right afferent pupillary defect, and right optic disk edema.

27. _____ Diagnostic possibilities include:

    A. Vertebral artery dissection
    B. Cervical radiculopathy
    C. Demyelinating disorder
    D. Subacute combined system disease
    E. None of the above

28. _____ Diagnostic studies most sensitive to detect the underlying neurological disorder include:

    A. LP
    B. NCV-EMG
    C. Spinal cord somatosensory potentials
    D. Cervical MRI
    E. Brain MRI

29. _____ If T-2 MRI shows one high-signal-intensity lesion in the cervical spinal cord, the diagnosis is most likely:

    A. Transverse myelitis
    B. Multiple sclerosis
    C. Glioma
    D. Meningioma
    E. None of the above

30. _____ Factors which may cause multiple sclerosis:

    A. Stress
    B. Pregnancy
    C. Trauma
    D. Diet
    E. None of the above

RESPONSES AND EXPLANATIONS

1. **T.** The diagnosis of MS is established on a clinical basis and may be supported or confirmed by laboratory neurodiagnostic studies. There should be two or more discrete clinical episodes. The neurological findings should be located in physically *noncontiguous* regions, e.g., optic neuritis and thoracic transverse myelitis, to confirm to spatial dissemination. *(Neurologic Clinics of North America 13, pp. 119–146, 1995; Ref. 1, pp. 811–816; Ref. 2, pp. 653–655)*

2. **T.** Fatigue is a major disabling feature in MS patients; however, the patient must have clinical symptoms and signs which confirm the diagnosis of MS. Do not confuse MS with chronic fatigue syndrome or fibromyalgia. For example, if the patient reports the symptom of fatigue and has normal neurological examination, this is not likely to be MS. *(Ref. 1, pp. 814, 824; Ref. 2, pp. 718–719)*

3. **F.** Neck flexion can cause electrical paresthesias which extend down the back to the thighs and legs (Lhermitte sign). This occurs in demyelination involving posterior columns of the cervical spinal cord. This is seen in multiple sclerosis, spondylitic cervical myelopathy, and subacute combined system disease. *(Ref. 1, pp. 27, 488, 814; Ref. 2, pp. 160, 654)*

4. **F.** Seizures and cognitive decline are cortical gray-matter manifestations and are *uncommon* in MS. Behavioral disturbances such as depression are common in MS, and the emotional lability of pseudobulbar palsy is frequently seen in MS (although pseudobulbar palsy is seen with other neurological conditions including bilateral strokes). *(Ref. 1, pp. 811–815; Ref. 2, pp. 653–656)*

5. **T.** Heat worsens CNS electrical synaptic conduction in MS patients. This formed the basis for the "hot bath" test. Patients with suspected MS were placed in a "hot bath" to determine if clinical manifestations worsened or new symptoms developed. This test is rarely utilized now, as there were occasional patients who went blind due to optic neuritis which developed when they were placed in a "hot bath." MS patients report worsening of symptoms and increased fatigue during the "dog days of summer." *(Ref. 2, pp. 178, 180)*

6. **T.** The presence of high-signal-intensity lesions on T-2 weighted image suggests the diagnosis of MS. Noncontrast MRI findings tell *nothing* regarding disease activity. If T-1 MRI shows that the lesion enhances following administration of paramagnetic contrast agent (gadolinium), this indicates *active* MS. *(Neurologic Clinics of North America 13, p. 147, 1995; Ref. 1, pp. 815–820; Ref. 2, pp. 657–661; Ref. 5, pp. 490–493)*

7. **T.** MS is more common in temperate than in tropical areas. Northern Europe and the United States are areas of high prevalence, whereas southern Europe and Africa are low-prevalence areas. Geographic latitude and race are independent risk factors (Asians and Blacks have low risk). *(Ref. 1, pp. 804–809; Ref. 2, pp. 653–655)*

8. **T.** In MS, there is an immunological attack against the CNS. Inflammatory cells (T-4 and T-8 lymphocytes) are found within the acute lesions, and these result in myelin destruction. Since oligodendrocytes are responsible for myelin formation in the CNS (Schwann cells are responsible in the peripheral nervous system), there is evidence that they are injured in MS. The axons are relatively spared in MS. With time, active MS lesions become inactive acellular demyelinated plaques. *(Neurologic Clinics of North America 13, p. 51, 1995; Ref. 1, pp. 805–806; Ref. 2, pp. 655–656)*

9. **T.** Fatigue may be alleviated by amantadine and pemoline; however, their effect is usually temporary. Also, fatigue is best avoided by a change in work schedule. Fatigue may be a prominent symptom of depression. *(Ref. 1, pp. 822–824; Ref. 2, pp. 662–663)*

10. **T.** MS rarely causes pain; however, isolated single pontine plaque may cause trigeminal neuralgia. Sensory loss and paresthesias are common neurological disturbances due to MS. *(Ref. 1, p. 813)*

11. **T.** The primary lesion in MS is loss of CNS myelin. This is followed by development of acellular *plaque. (Ref. 1, pp. 807–811; Ref. 2, p. 657)*

12. **T.** For an acute attack of optic neuritis or transverse myelitis, utilize high-dose intravenous methylprednisolone for 7 days, followed by a tapering schedule of oral prednisone for 4 weeks. Chronic oral corticosteroids do not alter the course of MS. There is no evidence for proven efficacy of immunosuppression. Interferon is established therapy for exacerbating-remitting MS and possibly chronic progressive MS (studies in progress). *(Neurologic Clinics of North America 13, p. 173, 1995; Ref. 1, pp. 822–823; Ref. 2, p. 663)*

13. **B**
14. **E**
15. **D**
16. **A**
17. **C**

13–17. Neuromyelitis optica is a transverse or ascending myelitis followed or preceded by acute or subacute blindness in one or both eyes. This represents the fulminant form of MS, but the pathology is similar to that of other forms. PML is a demyelinating disorder caused by papovavirus. It is seen most commonly in immunosuppressed patients, e.g., AIDS and transplant patients. It begins with subcortical demyelination in the parietal-occipital cortex, and these lesions may cause visual hallucinations. Transverse myelitis may follow an initial viral illness and cause motor, sensory, and autonomic disturbances, usually involving both legs. This demyelination usually begins in the midthoracic region but may develop at any level. Bilateral INO is most commonly due to a medial longitudinal fasciculus lesion due to medial pontine demyelination. INO can be caused by other primary brainstem lesions, e.g., pontine glioma. Charcot triad (scanning speech, tremor, gait ataxia) is due to posterior fossa (cerebellar, brainstem) demyelination. *(Ref. 1, pp. 811–814, 825–826; Ref. 2, pp. 454, 572)*

18. **E.** The clinical course of MS may vary. Rarely, cases are clinically silent and are detected by MRI or necropsy findings only. Some patients have a benign course with few, mild exacerbations and complete remissions. Good prognosis is expected if there is minimal disability 5 years after initial onset of symptoms or if initial symptoms are predominantly sensory. *(Neurologic Clinics of North America 13, p. 119, 1995; Ref. 1, pp. 821–822)*

19. **E.** Elevated CSF gamma-globulin is seen in all listed conditions. Myelin basic protein, oligoclonal immunoglobulin bands, and increased intrathecal gamma-globulin are relatively specific CSF findings for MS. *(Ref. 1, pp. 815–816; Ref. 2, p. 657)*

20. **A.** Interferon reduces exacerbation rate in relapsing-remitting MS as well as reducing the number of MRI lesions. Interferon has not yet been shown to be effective in progressive MS. *(Ref. 1, p. 822–823)*

21. **B.** MRI is the most sensitive diagnostic study for MS. It shows high-signal-intensity lesions on T-2 weighted image and low-signal-intensity lesions on T-1 weighted image. The latter may show *enhancement* after gadolinium administration. Lesions in the corpus callosum, brainstem and cerebellum, and the periventricular region are common in MS; however, these are not *specific*. Remember, diagnosis of MS is clinically based and *not* established by any laboratory studies. *(Neurologic Clinics of North America 13, p. 147, 1995; Ref. 1, pp. 815–818)*

22. **D.** Transverse myelitis is usually of viral or postinfectious origin but may also occur following immunizations. There is sudden onset of motor, sensory, and autonomic dysfunction. Due to the initial stage of "spinal shock," reflexes are absent; several days to weeks later, hyperreflexia develops. The sensory disturbance localizes the lesion to the midthoracic region. The course is variable; however, recovery frequently occurs within 2–8 weeks. This is usually a *monophasic* illness, but in some instances MS may develop later. The lack of visual disturbances indicates that this is not Devic disease. The lack of *back pain* is against neoplasm or abscess. *(Ref. 2, pp. 598–599; Ref. 5, p. 468)*

23. **D.** To exclude all other possible clinical conditions, these diagnostic studies should be performed. If myelin basic protein or oligoclonal bands are present, this suggests MS. MRI is negative in most cases of transverse myelitis, but it may occasionally show cord swelling and high-signal-intensity lesions in the mid-thoracic region. When this abnormality occurs, lesions *disappear* with time. MRI is more likely to fail to show *spinal* than brain lesions in MS patients. *(Ref. 1, pp. 815–816; Ref. 2, p. 657)*

24. **E.** All of these listed laboratory tests might *suggest* MS. They would *not* confirm the diagnosis of MS because clinical manifestations are *monophasic*, without dissemination in time and space. This course is not consistent with MS. *(Ref. 2, pp. 598–600)*

25. **A.** Because of presumed immunological reaction and cord swelling, most patients are treated with high-dose intravenous methylprednisolone; however, there is no evidence that this is effective unless acute transverse myelitis is due to MS. The other listed treatments have been utilized for MS. *(Ref. 2, p. 600)*

26. **E.** If *brain* MRI shows multiple periventricular lesions, this *suggests* the possibility of MS; however, other listed conditions may cause multiple brain and spinal cord lesions. Since other conditions represent systemic disorders, full evaluation is warranted. *(Ref. 1, pp. 819–820)*

27. **C.** The combination of spinal cord plus optic nerve findings suggests MS. The pattern could be seen in combined system disease, but sudden onset is not consistent with B_{12} deficiency. The occurrence of neurological dysfunction following neck trauma should raise the possibility of vertebral artery dissection or cervical radiculopathy; however, the listed neurological disturbances do not suggest either disorder. *(Ref. 1, pp. 819–820)*

28. **E.** With clinical features suggesting spinal cord and optic nerve demyelination, brain MRI is most sensitive. LP with CSF examination is more specific but less sensitive for detecting MS. If cervical myelopathy or radiculopathy is suspected, cervical MRI should be performed. *(Ref. 1, pp. 816, 820)*

29. **B.** Even if MRI shows only spinal cord lesions, MS is the most likely diagnosis. Transverse myelitis due to spinal demyelination explains the motor and sensory abnormalities; however, the eye findings suggest optic neuritis. *(Ref. 2, pp. 664–665)*

30. **E.** None of these factors *causes* MS, but stress (emotional, physical) or physical injury may *precipitate* MS in any individual who is already immunologically and genetically predisposed. In this case, physical trauma may have precipitated the initial MS attack; however, this sequence is controversial and not supported by clinical studies. *(Ref. 1, pp. 804–808)*

20

CHILDHOOD NEUROLOGICAL DISORDERS

Matching

Match the clinical features with the childhood seizure type.

A. Brief generalized major motor seizure precipitated when the patient's body temperature rises

B. Brief staring episodes; eyelids blink rhythmically; 3-cps spike-and-wave EEG pattern

C. Nocturnal seizures; usually resolve by age 14; EEG shows bilateral spike discharge in central temporal region

D. Rapid flexor spasms; commonly occur in patients with tuberous sclerosis

E. May simulate jitteriness of newborn; difficult to recognize due to fragmentary seizure pattern; may be due to metabolic disorder

1. _____ Petit mal

2. _____ Febrile

3. _____ Benign Rolandic

4. _____ Infantile spasms

5. _____ Neonatal

Match the metabolic disorder with the neurological condition.

A. Hexosaminidase A deficiency

B. Abnormal long-chain fatty acids

C. Arylsulfatase A deficiency

D. Dystrophin abnormality

E. Defect in branched-chain amino acid metabolism

F. Alpha-glucosidase deficiency

6. _____ Metachromatic leukodystrophy (MLD)

7. _____ Duchenne muscular dystrophy

8. _____ Maple syrup urine disease (MSUD)

9. _____ Pompe's disease

10. _____ Adrenoleukodystrophy

11. _____ Tay-Sachs disease

Match the clinical feature with the neurological disorder.

A. Bilateral acoustic neuromas; Lisch nodules

B. Adenoma sebaceum; seizures; mental retardation

C. Port-wine nevus of face; intracranial calcifications

D. Ataxia; absent reflexes; impaired proprioception

E. Spasticity; peripheral neuropathy; blindness

12. _____ Metachromatic leukodystrophy (MLD)

13. _____ Tuberous sclerosis (TS)

14. _____ Sturge-Weber syndrome (SWS)

15. _____ Friedreich's ataxia (FA)

16. _____ Neurofibromatosis (NF)

Match the nervous system malformation with the characteristic features.

A. Myelomeningocele

B. Spina bifida occulta

C. Holoprosencephaly

D. Microcephaly

E. Polymicrogyria

F. Pachygyria

G. Agenesis of corpus callosum

17. _____ Failure of cerebral hemispheric fiber connections

18. _____ Multiple small poorly formed gyri of cerebral hemispheres

19. _____ Head circumference which is greater than two standard deviations below mean

20. _____ Poor neuron migration with thicker than normal gray matter

21. _____ Forebrain does not divide into two hemispheres and there is a single ventricle

22. _____ Incomplete formation of vertebral bodies

23. _____ Defect in which spinal cord and meninges protrude through bone defect

Match the clinical features with the neurological condition.

A. Rapidly progressive form of infantile hypotonic quadriplegia

B. Cause of mild proximal weakness

C. Cause of transient weakness in newborn

D. Severe weakness and associated cardiomyopathy

E. Associated with muscle stiffness and cataracts

24. _____ Kugelberg-Welander disease

25. _____ Werdnig-Hoffmann disease

26. _____ Duchenne dystrophy

27. _____ Myotonic dystrophy

28. _____ Neonatal myasthenia gravis

Match the clinical feature with the neurological condition.

A. Pseudohypertrophy

B. Positive Gowers sign

C. Unilateral shoulder weakness

D. Weakness of one hand and Horner syndrome

E. Bilateral foot drop

29. _____ Charcot-Marie-Tooth (CMT)

30. _____ Limb-girdle dystrophy

31. _____ Erb-Duchenne paralysis

32. _____ Klumpke paralysis

33. _____ Duchenne muscular dystrophy

Multiple Choice

Choose the most appropriate response.

34. _____ At 24 months, a normal child should be able to:

A. Feed self
B. Point to objects
C. Run
D. Talk in 2- to 3-word sentences
E. All of the above

35. _____ Cerebral palsy most commonly occurs in:

A. Diabetic mothers
B. Low-birth-weight infants
C. If kernicterus has occurred
D. Both A and B
E. Both B and C

36. _____ Clinical features of perinatal hypoxic-ischemic encephalopathy include:

A. Neuropathy
B. Myopathy
C. Psychoses
D. Chorea-athetosis
E. Brachial plexus dysfunction

37. _____ Manifestations of Von Hippel-Lindau disease include:

A. Hemangioblastoma of cerebellum and retina
B. Renal cyst
C. Pheochromocytoma
D. All of the above
E. None of the above

H.R. is a 30- year-old white male with type II vonRecklinghausen disease on his maternal side. He has *no* skin lesions. He develops difficulty understanding telephone conversations but has normal hearing tests.

38. _____ Which of the following is (are) true:

A. It is unlikely that he has this neurocutaneous disorder
B. It is likely that he is anxious but has no neurological disorder
C. Consider acoustic neuroma as explanation of symptoms
D. Consider presbyacusis as cause of hearing symptoms
E. Both A and B

39. _____ Clinical features of vitamin E deficiency include:

A. Seizures
B. Mental retardation
C. Spinocerebellar degeneration
D. Intracranial hypertension
E. All of the above

40. _____ The vascular lesion in Moyamoya disease involves:

A. Occlusion of internal carotid artery with extensive collateral pattern
B. Carotid artery dissection
C. Lenticulostriate occlusion
D. Basilar artery occlusion
E. Anterior spinal artery occlusion

41. _____ The major drawback to phenobarbital therapy in children is:

A. Ataxia
B. Hyperactivity
C. Hirsutism
D. Liver toxicity
E. Bone marrow suppression

42. _____ The major drawback to phenytoin therapy in adolescent patients, leading to noncompliance and poor seizure control, might be:

A. Hirsutism and gingival hyperplasia
B. Ataxia
C. Hepatotoxicity
D. Renal toxicity
E. Peripheral neuropathy

43. _____ The following is true of craniopharyngioma:

A. Arise from pituitary fossa
B. Cause bitemporal inferior quadrantanopsia
C. Invade cavernous sinus
D. Cause acromegaly
E. Radioresponsive tumor

44. _____ The following is true of pineal tumors:

A. Cause Parinaud syndrome
B. Arise from pituitary fossa
C. Cause bitemporal hemianopsia
D. Cause centrocecal scotoma
E. Cause seizures

45. _____ The following is (are) associated with ataxia-telangiectasia:

A. Skin and conjunctival lesions
B. Chorea-athetosis

C. Sino-pulmonary infections
D. Lymphoreticular neoplasms
E. All of the above

46. _____ This is true of Sydenham's chorea:

A. There is always clinical evidence of prior streptococcal infection
B. Clinical heart disease is always present
C. Seizures are commonly present
D. Fidgetiness, clumsiness, and facial dyskinesias are common features
E. Hemiparesis and spasticity are common features

47. _____ Clinical features of lead toxicity include:

A. Wrist drop
B. Convulsions
C. Anemia
D. Intracranial hypertension
E. All of the above

48. _____ In patients with cerebellar astrocytomas:

A. Seizures are common
B. Dementia is an early sign
C. Intracranial calcification are common
D. Papilledema and diplopia may be early signs
E. Cystic tumors are uncommon

49. _____ Clinical features of pontine gliomas include:

A. Diplopia
B. Ataxia
C. Bifacial paresis
D. Pyramidal tract signs
E. All of the above

50. _____ Complications of bacterial meningitis in children include:

A. Subdural effusion
B. Cerebral infarction
C. Hearing loss
D. Hydrocephalus
E. All of the above

51. _____ Common congenital infections of the CNS include:

A. Rubella
B. Toxoplasmosis
C. Cytomegalovirus
D. Herpes simplex
E. All of the above

RESPONSES AND EXPLANATIONS

1. **B.** Absence seizures are characterized by brief confusional episodes in which the child appears to be day-dreaming. There is no aura and no postictal confusion. EEG shows characteristic 3-cps spike-and-wave activity. Treat with valproic acid. *(Ref. 2, pp. 329–330; Ref. 4, pp. 164–165)*

2. **A.** Seizures of generalized major motor type which occur on the ascending limb of a temperature curve may be prevented with phenobarbital, but this is not usually needed. A rectal form of diazepam is being developed for treatment (it is not yet approved in the United States). *(Ref. 2, pp. 338, 391)*

3. **C.** Centrotemporal seizures are benign focal seizures which usually occur at night. They respond to phenytoin or carbamazepine and cease spontaneously in adolescence. *(Ref. 2, p. 392)*

4. **D.** These begin in children between 3 and 12 months of age. They consist of sudden brief flexor spasms of the head, neck, trunk, and extremities. Each episode lasts only seconds. EEG shows diffuse, irregular, high-voltage slow waves with interspersed spikes. They are frequently associated with major congenital or developmental brain abnormalities. *(Ref. 2, pp. 336, 393–395)*

5. **E.** The most common causes are asphyxia (hypoxic-ischemic encephalopathy) or infection (sepsis, bacterial meningitis). Hemorrhage and developmental anomalies also cause neonatal seizures. They begin within 24 hr of birth. Also, common metabolic factors (hypoglycemia, hypocalcemia, narcotic withdrawal syndrome of addicted mothers) may precipitate these seizures. Phenobarbital is the best AED to utilize in the neonatal period. *(Ref. 2, pp. 394–395)*

6. **C.** MLD is due to arylsulfatase A deficiency. There is diffuse central and peripheral nervous system demyelination with accumulation of metachromatic granules. Clinical features of white-matter demyelination (gait disorder, weakness, spasticity, increased reflexes, Babinski signs, optic atrophy) and peripheral neuropathy may develop. *(Ref. 1, pp. 558–560)*

7. **D.** This is a sex-linked recessive disorder due to the absence of the muscle protein *dystrophin*, which is a component of the muscle cytoskeleton. *(Ref. 2, pp. 507–510)*

8. **E.** MSUD is due to a defect in branched-chain amino acids and is characterized by urine that smells like maple syrup. There is a defect in oxidative decarboxylation of branch-chained keto-acids. Clinically, there are episodes of abnormal respiration and muscle tone, followed by progressive neurological deterioration. Diagnosis is established by positive dinitrophenylhydrazine test. *(Ref. 1, pp. 538–555)*

9. **F.** Pompe's disease is type II glycogenosis which causes glycogen accumulation in *lysosomes* of skeletal muscle, heart, liver, and brain. Lysosomal acid alpha-glucosidase is deficient. Clinical manifestations are muscle weakness and impaired cardiac function. *(Ref. 1, pp. 572–574)*

10. **B.** This disorder is characterized by visual loss, dementia, spasticity, and seizures. It is sex-linked recessive and occurs with adrenocortical deficiency. There is diffuse demyelination of cerebral white matter. There is accumulation of long-chain fatty acids in white-matter cholesterol esters. *(Ref. 1, pp. 560–561)*

11. **A.** Tay-Sachs is GM_2 gangliosidosis in which this substance accumulates in brain gray matter. It is due to a defect in hexosaminidase activity. Clinical features include intellectual deterioration, hypotonia, and presence of a retinal cherry-red spot. *(Ref. 1, pp. 550–551)*

12. **E.** MLD causes *central* demyelination leading to spasticity, optic atrophy, Babinski signs, and evidence of peripheral demyelination (absent reflexes, reduced sensation in distal distribution). *(Ref. 1, pp. 558–560)*

13. **B.** TS is a neurocutaneous syndrome (phakomatoses) in which tubers (gliotic areas) develop within the CNS and myelination is reduced. Clinical features include mental retardation, seizures, adenoma sebaceum, and tumors in multiple organs including the CNS. *(Ref. 1, pp. 640–647; Ref. 2, pp. 401–402)*

14. **C.** In SWS, there is port-wine vascular nevus in the ophthalmic region of the trigeminal nerve (upper face), contralateral focal seizures, and intracranial (usually occipital) calcifications. There is leptomeningeal angiomatosis in the parieto-occipital region. *(Ref. 1, pp. 635–638; Ref. 2, pp. 402–403)*

15. **D.** FA is spinocerebellar ataxia characterized by ataxia, nystagmus, kyphoscoliosis, pes cavus, proprioceptive disturbance, and Babinski signs. The primary lesion involves ascending and descending spinal cord tracts and cerebellum. *(Ref. 1, pp. 686–688; Ref. 2, pp. 461–462)*

16. **A.** NF (von Recklinghausen's disease) is separated into two genetically different forms—type I and type II. Type I has peripheral manifestations and type II has central manifestations. In type I there are multiple tumors within the central and peripheral nervous systems, with prominent cutaneous lesions (*cafe au lait* spots, freckling). Nodules may develop with iris (Lisch nodules). Intracranial (optic, acoustic) tumors may also develop. *(Ref. 1, p. 630; Ref. 2, pp. 398–400)*

17. **G.** This may be partial or complete. It may be associated with micropolygyria, cortical heterotopia of gray matter, and Dandy-Walker syndrome. *(Ref. 1, pp. 517–532)*

18. **E.** This results in cerebral gyri which are too small and too numerous. There is defective cellular lamination. This causes mental retardation, spasticity, and hypotonia. *(Ref. 1, pp. 517–532)*

19. **D.** This must consider age, race, and sex. Microcephaly usually reflects the presence of small underlying brain. It may be primary due to developmental anomalies or secondary to brain injury.

20. **F.** Pachygyria (macrogyria) is associated with a gyral pattern that is too coarse and too few such that the gray matter region is thickened. There are areas of focal cortical dysplasia which may lead to seizures. *(Ref. 1, pp. 517–522)*

21. **C.** This is an anterior midline defect in which the primary cerebral vesicle fails to cleave and there is a single ventricular cavity. There are associated midline facial defects. *(Ref. 1, pp. 517–520)*

22. **B.** This is failure of fusion of the posterior vertebral arches. There is no herniation of meninges or neural tissue. The skin of the back is normal. *(Ref. 2, p. 396)*

23. **A.** Meningocele is herniation of meninges through defective posterior arches, but in myelomeningocele neural tissue protrudes. It is possible to differentiate these two conditions when they are surgically repaired. *(Ref. 2, p. 396)*

24. **B.** This is a milder form of spinal muscle atrophy in which patients initially develop *proximal* muscle weakness (unusual, as most other motor neuron diseases begin *distally*). Weakness may not develop until adult life, and there may be slow worsening. *(Ref. 2, pp. 147, 492)*

25. **A.** This is spinal muscular atrophy which occurs in infancy or early childhood. It is manifested by widespread muscular weakness and atrophy. Motor neurons of the brainstem may be affected, causing swallowing and respiratory difficulties. Diagnosis is established by EMG and muscle biopsy findings. *(Ref. 1, pp. 505, 743; Ref. 2, pp. 491–492)*

26. **D.** This disorder affects *skeletal* and cardiac muscle. Patients may die of respiratory insufficiency or cardiac failure. *(Ref. 2, pp. 507–510)*

27. **E.** This is inherited as autosomal dominant, with the abnormality situated on chromosome 19. Initial weakness is *distal,* with prominent myotonia (failure to relax muscle such that patients report "stiffness"). *(Ref. 2, pp. 515–517; Ref. 4, pp. 232–233)*

28. **C.** This is a transient disorder which occurs in 15% of infants born to myasthenic mothers. Symptoms begin within 24 hr of birth. The infant has poor cry and suck, and muscles appear hypotonic. Antibody titers to acetylcholine receptor are elevated. Treat with anticholinesterase medication. The disorder resolves spontaneously within 6 weeks . This is a different disorder than congenital MG, which does not resolve and does not develop as early as transient MG. *(Ref. 1, p. 755)*

29. **E.** CMT is a hereditary motor and sensory polyneuropathy. Symptoms begin in the first or second decade. Atrophy of distal legs leads to "stork leg" deformity. Foot deformities including pes cavus (flat feet) are common. EMG shows marked slowing of nerve conduction velocities due to demyelinating neuropathy. *(Ref. 1, pp. 652–655; Ref. 2, pp. 484–486)*

30. **B.** In limb-girdle dystrophy, there is proximal muscle weakness which initially begins in the pelvic girdle. Arising from the floor without using the hands for support is very difficult, and patients use their arms to push up (positive Gowers sign). *(Ref. 2, pp. 506, 511)*

31. **C.** Perinatal injury to the upper portion of the brachial plexus is referred to as Erb-Duchenne paralysis. This is usually unilateral. The shoulder is adducted and internally rotated, the elbow is extended, the forearm is pronated, and the wrist is flexed. *(Ref. 1, p. 477)*

32. **D.** Klumpke paralysis is isolated paralysis of the lower portion of the brachial plexus. Paralysis involves intrinsic hand muscles with weakness of the flexors of wrist and fingers. There may be unilateral Horner syndrome due to involvement of cervical sympathetic fibers. *(Ref. 1, p. 477)*

33. **A.** In Duchenne muscular dystrophy, calf muscles are weak but show *pseudohypertrophy.* Calves are enlarged and have rubbery consistency as a result of infiltration and replacement of muscle fibers by fat and connective tissue. *(Ref. 2, pp. 507–510)*

34. **E.** At 24 months, a child should have begun to talk in short sentences. Running capability is clumsy, but the child should have normal motor and coordination capability. *(Ref. 1, pp. 507–512)*

35. **E.** Risk factors for hypoxic-ischemic brain injury (cerebral palsy) include kernicterus (neonatal jaundice), low birth weight, and prematurity. Remember, these patients may have no paralysis or mental retardation; however, spastic diplegia or spastic hemiplegia are the most common clinical manifestations. *(Ref. 1, pp. 507–511)*

36. **D.** In cerebral palsy, mental retardation, seizures, and motor deficit are most common. Chorea, athetosis, and cerebellar dysfunction may result. Brachial plexus lesion results from physical trauma during birth. *(Ref. 1, pp. 507–511)*

37. **D.** In von Hippel-Lindau syndrome, cerebellar and spinal cord hemangioblastoma occur with associated pancreatic cysts,

and kidney and adrenal tumors. Angiomas may be seen in the retina. Diagnosis of cerebellar lesion is established by characteristic CT/MRI and angiographic findings. *(Ref. 1, pp. 338, 385)*

38. **C.** These patients may have bilateral acoustic neuromas. These cause retrocochlear hearing loss in which word discrimination is quite poor despite minimal hearing loss. This poor speech discrimination may be noted while talking on the telephone or while listening to conversation in a noisy room. *(Ref. 1, pp. 326–328)*

39. **C.** Vitamin E deficiency (tocopherol) may occur in malabsorption syndromes and cystic fibrosis. Patients may develop spinocerebellar degeneration and neuropathy. *(Ref. 1, pp. 949–950)*

40. **A.** Arterial occlusion in childhood is uncommon. Angiography is needed when acute hemiplegia develops to establish the underlying vascular cause of the stroke. Moyamoya's disease is arteriopathy with narrowing of basal carotid arteries with dilatation of major cerebral arteries and prominent collateral circulation. *(Ref. 1, pp. 267–268)*

41. **B.** Hyperactivity, inattention, and cognitive slowing are major drawbacks to phenobarbital. This is otherwise a very safe drug with minimal systemic toxicity. *(Ref. 2, pp. 322–323, 326, 344)*

42. **A.** Cosmetic effects on gums and skin with hirsutism are reasons adolescents become noncompliant with phenytoin. Physicians underestimate noncompliance by 50% in seizure patients taking *any* AED. *(Ref. 2, pp. 322–323)*

43. **B.** Craniopharyngiomas are suprasellar calcified cystic tumors. They cause bitemporal hemianopsia which *initially* appears as *inferior* quadrantanopsia. Also, it causes hypopituitarism, not pituitary hyperfunction. *(Ref. 2, pp. 436–437)*

44. **A.** Pineal tumors predominantly affect boys. Early signs include Parinaud syndrome (paralysis of conjugate upward gaze, dilated pupils with impaired light reaction) and increased intracranial pressure. *(Ref. 2, pp. 437–439)*

45. **E.** In this disorder, there is cerebellar ataxia, chorea-athetosis, conjunctival and skin telangiectasia, susceptibility to sinus-pulmonary infection, and lymphoma. The gene for this disorder is localized to chromosome 11. *(Ref. 1, pp. 691–693)*

46. **D.** The major neurological manifestation of rheumatic fever is *chorea.* Involuntary movements involve the face, hands, and arms. The patient may be clumsy and fidgety. Chorea lasts 1–24 months and resolves after that time. This is a post-streptococcal complication, but the initial infection may not be detected or treated. It can be prevented by early treatment with penicillin. The chorea can be controlled with Haldol. *(Ref. 1, pp. 699–701)*

47. **E.** Lead may cause neuropathy leading to wrist drop. If the CNS is affected, intracranial hypertension and convulsions may occur. Anemia and renal tubular dysfunction may occur. Red blood cells show basophilic stippling. *(Ref. 1, pp. 990–991)*

48. **D.** Cerebellar astrocytomas are usually cystic tumors which compress the cerebellum and fourth ventricle. This results in obstructive hydrocephalus and ataxia. *(Ref. 1, pp. 338–340; Ref. 2, pp. 434–435)*

49. **E.** Pontine gliomas grow within the brainstem to cause all listed findings. Signs of intracranial hypertension develop late as this tumor infiltrates into the brainstem. *(Ref. 2, p 435)*

50. **E.** All are potential complications of meningitis in children. *H. influenza* is most likely to cause subdural effusion. Meningitis is a common cause of stroke in children. Cranial nerve dysfunction may lead to hearing impairment. Meningeal exudate may obstruct CSF pathways and result in hydrocephalus. *(Ref. 1, p. 111)*

51. **E.** All are potential *congenital* CNS problems which may lead to poor CNS development. Varicella is another virus which may affect the CNS. Mental retardation, eye disorders (cataract, glaucoma, chorioretinitis) and intracranial calcification may develop. *(Ref. 1, p. 499)*

T - #0707 - 101024 - C0 - 276/216/9 - PB - 9780876308684 - Gloss Lamination